ARTHRITIS AND COMMON SENSE
GOOD HEALTH AND COMMON SENSE
HEALTHY HAIR AND COMMON SENSE
COMMON COLD AND COMMON SENSE

# HEALTHY HAIR
## and
# COMMON SENSE
## by
# Dan Dale Alexander

THE WITKOWER PRESS, INC.

ILLUSTRATIONS BY JOYCE HURWITZ

*I wish to express my deepest thanks to Jack Matcha for his invaluable assistance in the preparation of this book.*

D.A.

# CONTENTS

# HEALTHY HAIR
## AND
# COMMON SENSE

# OFF TO A NEW HEAD START

If you are losing your hair, don't lose your head along with it. There *is* something you can do about it. I know—because something worked for me.

This book advances a new concept in treating the problem of hair loss—a revolutionary concept that can be regarded as a breakthrough in the stale and cluttered thinking that has surrounded the treatment of baldness for generations. It is based on thirty years of exploring the field, of searching for an answer that would help me.

After years of experimenting with various ways of stopping my own serious hair loss, I have found a way. It has stopped my hair from falling. It has arrested my own baldness. It has helped me to grow wonderful new hair. I have every reason to believe that it will help you.

1

# CROSS SECTION OF THE SCALP

There is infinitely more to the hair than meets the eye, as this cross section readily demonstrates. Do not be deceived, however, by its resemblance to a hero sandwich. The magnification is great and the apparently vast distance between the diploe (the skull) and the point on the scalp where the hair shaft emerges can best be reduced to reality by putting your finger on your scalp and feeling the skull beneath. It would be well to study this drawing carefully in order to understand various related references in the text and in other illustrations.

The various sections shown are:

*The Epidermis*—The outer layer of the scalp.

*The Hair Shaft*—The life of which is a concern of all of us, it is surrounded by the hair follicle, a small pocket pushing into the skin from the surface, at the bottom of which is a cluster of cells, called the *Matrix*, from which the hair grows.

*The Sebaceous Gland*—One of the skin glands, which secrete oily matter for lubrication of hair and skin.

*The Matrix*—A cluster of cells from which the hair grows. This matrix, in the human scalp, will produce on the average of 0.355mm, a little more than one-hundredth of an inch, of hair per day.

*The Hair Bulb*—The base of the hair follicle which surrounds the actual hair shaft. It has a hole filled with connective tissue, which is called...

*The Dermal Papilla*—A compact group of blood vessels supplying nourishment to the hair root.

*The Fat Layer.*

*The Epicranial Aponeurosis*—The flattened tendon between the two fleshy bellies of the occipito-frontalis muscle (not shown).

*Connective Tissue*—The thin fibrous tissue called *Areolar Tisue*, which allows for movement of the upper scalp.

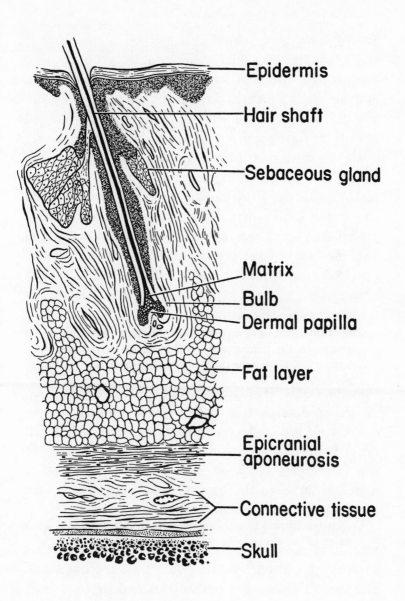

Epidermis

Hair shaft

Sebaceous gland

Matrix

Bulb

Dermal papilla

Fat layer

Epicranial aponeurosis

Connective tissue

Skull

The basic idea behind this method is not new. It was advanced over fifty years ago by a doctor who studied hair problems for years in clinics, universities, and hospitals in Paris, London, Vienna, and Berlin. He did not have the whole answer, but he learned enough to start scientists thinking along a new track.

He learned that hair must be nourished by the proper diet in order to grow and flourish. If our researchers in the field of hair problems had followed the lead of Dr. Richard W. Muller, our entire attitude toward the problems of dandruff, falling hair, and baldness might have been revolutionized. Millions of personal tragedies might have been averted. Unfortunately, Dr. Muller's work was ignored. But that's water over the dam. It is not the first time—nor will it be the last—that an important new idea in the field of scientific thinking has been brushed aside for decades.

What is important for me—and I believe for you—is that the book Dr. Muller wrote opened a new door. By going through that door, I have learned how to check hair loss and even how to regrow hair. I can never regrow all my hair, but I can regrow what I have lost in the past five years. I have done what no other man has done, to the best of my knowledge—I have regrown hair on a scheduled program.

I will explain all this in this book. I will tell you what foods to eat to nourish your hair and what foods to avoid. I will tell you how you must prepare them. But to get the most out of this book and its program, I think you should know a good deal more about hair

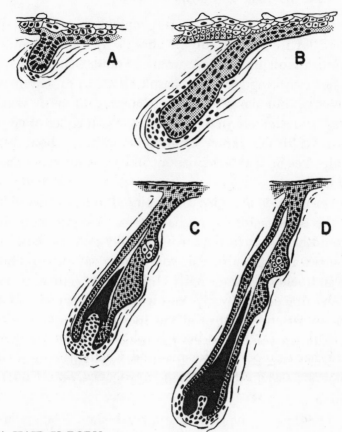

## A HAIR IS BORN

*A.* The hair germ stage.

*B.* Ectodermal (outer germ layer) downgrowth, leading to the hair growth stage.

*C.* Beginning of the formation of the papilla. The papilla is a small group of blood vessels at the root of the hair. The hair root is nourished by the arteries that bring new cleansed blood to this papilla.

*D.* Sheathed hair stage. The hair shaft now makes a definite appearance. A hair is born.

and its problems than most people know. Take my word for it, this is a subject about which most people know almost nothing. A woman knows that her hair is her crowning glory but hasn't a clue as to why it is thinning out dangerously or changing color. A man may be extremely well versed in the principles of general health but know absolutely nothing about his scalp. Yet he may worry about its condition every day of his life.

Perhaps you are a bit disappointed to learn that diet is the chief factor in my hair restoration program. It would be so much simpler if I merely told you how to concoct a magic salve that you rub on your scalp—and lo and behold, instant hair! Unfortunately, there is no such miraculous remedy. You will have to expend time and effort and, most of all, willpower. If it's any consolation to you, however, the same sensible diet that will improve the health of your hair will also improve your general health and enhance your sense of well-being.

The logic of the dietetic approach should be apparent to all. You accept the fact that, in a laboratory experiment, if a rat with a luxuriant growth of fur is put on a deficient diet its fur becomes lackluster and sparse and begins to fall out. When the rat is returned to a nourishing diet, the fur grows back in again.

Diet affects humans as well as rats. The catch is that those of us who have lost hair as a result of an impoverished diet did not undergo these changes dramatically; they happened so gradually that we did not relate cause with effect.

The chief task I set myself in this book, therefore, in addition to giving you solid information about the growth of hair that you cannot find in any other book except a medical text, is to analyze the many subtle differences between what most of us eat every day and what we should eat if we wish to follow the Dale Alexander method. It isn't simple and it isn't magic, as I pointed out before, but it worked for me and I see no reason why it shouldn't work for you.

## How One Book Led to Another

I felt compelled to write this book because of the many, many people who asked me to share my method with them. Some years ago I wrote a book called *Arthritis and Common Sense* in which I explained how certain dietary principles and oils help to alleviate the excruciating pain of arthritis. That book was bought by more than 750,000 persons in its original hardcover edition and was read by several million. Because of its impact on people, I received invitations to lecture on my method before groups in many states as well as in New Zealand and Australia. I appeared on numerous radio and television shows to explain how my program worked.

A curious thing began to happen as these lectures and appearances continued. When it comes to hair loss, I was an early bird, getting my start in high school. But during the period when I was lecturing, I began to lose hair much faster. Standing on a lecture platform naturally made me all the more self-conscious. After my lectures, many men in the same predicament, instead of asking me questions about arthritis, began to exchange opinions with me on our mutual problem of partial baldness. They told me stories of how they felt, rightly or wrongly, that their careers were hampered by baldness, how they had suffered acute embarrassment at parties and business meetings because they were teased about their patchy scalps. Not a few men were in constant torment lest girl friends or coworkers notice their hairpieces.

All of them had tried numerous oils, salves, scalp treatments. A few of them had even gone so far as to try hair transplantation by surgery to improve their appearances. Few were content with the results. Their hair loss still greatly disturbed them. Nearly all of them expressed the hope that someday somebody would write a book that would help them as much with that problem as *Arthritis and Common Sense* had helped in its area.

*Healthy Hair and Common Sense* is that book.

This book will tell you a great deal about the nature of hair and its problems that you probably don't know. You can, if you prefer, skip all this and go directly to my chapter on diet. After all, you need not know how aspirin works to know that it will stop your headache. But I think you'll follow the new method more intelligently and believe in it more firmly if you know the logic behind it.

So I hope you will read these chapters on hair and the story of my own trial-and-error search for the answer. At the end, I think you will understand why the new method helped my own serious falling hair and dandruff problem in a few weeks, and how it has started me on a wonderful cycle of regrowing hair that I had thought was beyond achievement. And you will understand why I firmly believe that this method will help you.

### An Apology to the Ladies

While I mention the problem of baldness among women here and there throughout this book, it is probably one of the most male-oriented books published since *Hunting the Great Alaskan Grizzly*. The reasons are pretty obvious. I'm a man, almost everyone with whom I've discussed the subject is a man, we tend to equate baldness almost exclusively with the male—plus a few other alibis I can't think of offhand. Nevertheless, thinning hair can also be a serious problem for women—in fact, increasingly so in recent years—and I owe those women afflicted with incipient or advanced loss of hair an apology for seeming to neglect the distaff side of the ledger.

True, many fewer women than men are afflicted. True, it's much easier for a woman than a man to disguise loss of hair. Still, to someone who is losing her hair, her problem is an acute one and calls for no less sympathy and concern than the man's, even though women's hair loss is much more a diffuse thinning and almost never progresses to total "billiard ball" type baldness.

I can only say in my defense that this book *is* written for women as well as for men. I go along with the French on their *vive la différence* philosophy, but it doesn't apply to diet, hair growth, and the other subjects with which this book is concerned. Therefore, whatever I say to men pertains equally to women.

I hope that women who read this book will accept my apology and my explanation and appreciate that no slight is intended. And I hope my seeming neglect will not prevent them from deriving whatever benefit this book may offer them.

And now, gentlemen and ladies—darn it, there I go again; will I never learn?—I mean, and now, ladies and gentlemen, let us apply ourselves to the *real* problem —the problem of hanging on to what hair you have left and striving to replenish some of the hair you've lost. Like all journeys, this one begins with a single step. And lo and behold! The very first chapter is entitled *That Big First Step.*

# 1

# THAT BIG FIRST STEP

I have never understood why hair, one of our greatest personal assets, is so neglected by both men and women. If our feet hurt, we go to a chiropodist. If our teeth ache, we see a dentist. But when we suffer from itchy, messy dandruff or see our hair fall out at an alarming rate, what do we do? We pour a Niagara of greasy kid stuff on our hair. Why? Because we've seen some television commercial for hair tonic or some technicolor magazine ad with a picture of a matinee idol boasting a full, glowing head of hair. When the magic tonic fails to do the job, we seek advice from friends or barbers. And when that fails we go in for wigs or toupees, paying hundreds of dollars to hide our embarrassment.

But that isn't the end of it. The new store-bought hairpiece, marvelously engineered and lifelike as it is, still leaves us insecure. We're afraid to go swimming or play tennis or dance one of the energetic new steps because the darned thing might fall off. We're afraid people will make fun of us as they've made fun of bald men since the prophet Elijah was mocked by little children.

Not long ago I went to see one of the most famous toupee manufacturers on the West Coast. He told me that not only has business zoomed in the past decade but that new types of customers were coming in.

In the old days, you could expect a good many actors and actresses to seek something to hide thinning locks or balding pates. It was natural enough under the circumstances. A performer makes his living by creating a certain public image. In the movies, on the stage, or on television, people expect him to look virile and handsome. A full, glowing head of hair is an important part of this image; and if he can't get his hair back any other way, a toupee is the final refuge.

But good hairpieces often cost several hundred dollars; you can't expect the average man or woman to order them. What is more, it is advisable to buy at least two, so that they can be kept clean and there is always a spare available.

Today, my informant tells me, he supplies many small business and professional men who, in the past, would never have considered wearing a hairpiece. The expense does not stop them.

Many come in because they're tired of being the butt of office jokes or nagging wives. Others are convinced that they will never get the right job or the long-sought promotion until they acquire that dashing, well-groomed look they've seen on the screen. What they don't realize is that, more often than not, that oversized screen hero is suffering from baldness himself and would give his last Cadillac to regrow his own hair.

Men wearing hairpieces may live in a constant state of embarrassment. Will the personnel manager raise an eyebrow during an interview for a new job? Will the potential customer stifle a giggle? Will the audience being addressed break out in a guffaw? Above all, will that new and fascinating young creature laugh out loud at a slight shift in the top-piece during a particularly intimate moment?

## An Alternative

Is there anyone wearing a toupee who would not be much happier if he could regrow his own hair? I've never met any such person in my thirty years of searching for an answer to baldness. And I myself am a happier and more contented man since I succeeded in regrowing my own hair. It has given me confidence and a sense of belonging that seems to enlarge my circle of friends—both men and women—to draw them closer to me, and give them, in turn, more confidence in me.

I emphasize the *three decades* of questioning and experimentation because I don't want you to think I achieved this success overnight. By much trial and error, I learned which foods were good for my hair and which were bad. I discovered how to make a specially formulated milk shake that became a key element in my hair-regrowth diet. I even learned through experiment that this special milk shake proved most effective when it was drunk on an empty stomach, as a substitute for breakfast.

Equally important, my long search showed me how to combat an inherited tendency toward baldness. I found the right combination of *germinating* foods, foods that nourish the "hair seed" that is responsible for the growth of new hair.

I have learned not only how to stop my hair loss but to regrow hair I have lost within the past five years. This is the true beginning—the long-awaited breakthrough. To my knowledge, no man before me has regrown hair on a *schedule*. It is this course of action, this *program*, that I want to pass on to you. If your hair is dry or thinning or your scalp itches or you suffer the annoyance of dandruff, you can profit from my experience.

My program doesn't depend on diet alone, nor on external stimulation or hair hygiene alone. All these and more will be discussed in detail in subsequent chapters. What to eat and what not to eat, how to massage the scalp, how and with what to shampoo your hair —these are the messages of this book, which I consider my chief endeavor, perhaps the culmination of my life's work.

## To Help Your Hair, Improve Your Blood

Blood is a living, growing thing. It consists of the fluid part, or plasma; the red blood cells, or corpuscles; and the white blood cells. The plasma carries the nutritive factors made from the food we eat to all tissues of the body, including the hair bulb—or "seed," in nonscientific language. It also carries certain minerals, especially sodium chloride, or common salt. The red blood cells carry oxygen, transmitted through the body in an oxygen-iron combination called oxyhemoglobin. They also carry potassium, a mineral essential to cell metabolism, and especially essential to the cells of the kidney tubules, where we rid ourselves of a large percentage of our bodily wastes.

The white cells can be thought of as scavengers that hurry to diseased or injured areas to encircle and pick up germs, dead tissues, and foreign bodies. The importance of healthy blood to the body functions in general and to the hair seeds in particular is readily apparent. In our program to grow healthy, robust, attractive hair, we will take advantage of these qualities of the blood. We will feed it the proper nutrients, confident that, as new red blood cells are formed continuously, about 1 percent being replaced daily, each one living about 120 days, and as the ingredients of the plasma and white cells are being renewed, we will be nourishing the hair seeds to the maximum.

If we add to the correct diet the correct massage, we

can bring more of the health-giving blood to the area where it is needed—the scalp. But any old massage won't do. There is a right and a wrong method here, too. In Chapter Twelve, I'll tell you all about it, in detail.

Healthy hair is formed from a great variety of ingredients and utilizes many complex chemicals in its luxuriant growth. These include oils, proteins, minerals, vitamins, enzymes, hormones, and other factors, known and unknown. Last but not least, there is one *magic ingredient*. It is my firm belief that this magic ingredient, which I shall describe in a later chapter, is of inestimable value in causing new hair to "sprout."

How do we transmit these invaluable nutrients to the hair? Through the bloodstream. And how do they get into the bloodstream? The basic ingredients must come from the food we eat, which is broken down by the digestive enzymes of the stomach and intestinal tract. From the intestinal tract these basic ingredients are picked up by the blood and carried to the liver, where some noxious materials are removed or modified. The purified blood then goes to the heart, to be pumped to the lungs to pick up life-giving oxygen. From there the oxygenated, enriched blood travels to all tissues of the body, to nourish and revivify every laggard cell, every recalcitrant organ. Provided—provided the blood contains the factors each particular organ needs. I learned by time-consuming and patient observation on myself which ingredients, when added

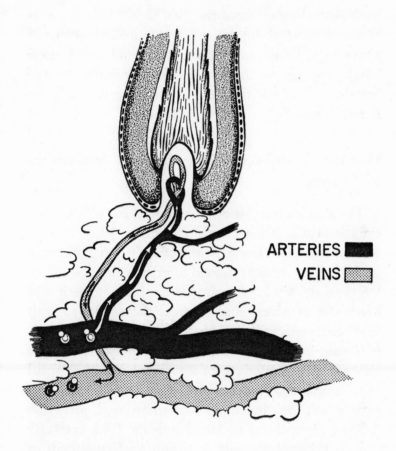

## HOW THE HAIR IS "FED"

The value of sound nutrition cannot be denied when one realizes that the arteries bring oxygenated and *nutritive* blood to the hair root while the veins carry away the wastes and carbon dioxide.

to the bloodstream from the diet, would help my hair bloom, and which ingredients would make it wither. I learned the importance of preparing and eating these foods properly, so that the hair seeds would get the benefit of full nourishment from these carefully selected foodstuffs.

### Why Has the Hair-Diet Relationship Been Unrecognized for So Long?

The reasons for this are manifold. First of all, if we eat a food that is not nourishing for the hair, or is actually harmful to the hair, the effect is not noticeable immediately, the way a food allergy is. If you are allergic to strawberries, you quickly begin to itch and break out in hives when you eat them. Not so with foods antagonistic to healthy hair growth. This effect is not an allergy. My experience shows that it takes about forty to sixty days for a constant diet of harmful food to manifest itself as dull hair or dandruff—and even longer for the hair to start thinning. Conversely, it takes about the same length of time for a carefully prepared diet of the most judiciously selected foods to add gloss and vigor to the "mane attraction." This is not an overnight result. But I strongly believe the long-range results will be worth the effort—many times over.

For example, I have found that ice cream is bad for the hair; yet it would take 90 to 180 consecutive days of consuming ice cream before its damage to the hair and scalp became noticeable. On the other hand, I have discovered that a raw, fertile egg, drunk in a specially formulated milk shake, is an excellent hair food. But, again, it would take 90 to 180 days of such drinks before the beneficial effects would be obvious. Originally, in preparing my research for this book, I referred to this as Alexander's Nutritive-Growth Cycle. I shall describe it more briefly, however, as the NuGrow Cycle.

On the average, hairs on the human scalp grow about 1/100 of an inch per day. If you were to eat a raw, fertile egg today, it would be fully digested within about twenty-four hours. Its nutritive components would find their way via the blood and lymph channels to the scalp and be incorporated in the growing hairs within another few hours. I believe that at least an inch of hair must grow on the male scalp, and perhaps an inch and a half to two inches on the female scalp, before the new healthy growth can be noticed.

As mentioned, I call this time from the intake of healthful food to its appearance as a new growth of healthy hair the NuGrow Cycle. This takes about 90 days in the male and about 180 days in the female. The difference stems not from any degree of faster hair growth in the male but from the fact that the short male haircut allows the change to be perceived sooner. It also means that one must stick to a diet of hair-nourishing foods and abstain from a diet of hair-harming foods for that length of time in order to see visible results. I don't mean to imply that one must be an absolute slave to such a regimen. An occasional ice cream soda, let's say one in two weeks, or skipping the

Hair Cocktail every so often, will probably produce no noticeable adverse effect. It is the continual consumption of sodas, candy, ice cream, and other sources of refined sugar and saturated fats that I consider the villain that foils your hair-raising adventure.

I trust I have made it clear that the long period that exists between ingestion and the effect of nutrients or toxins has obscured the relationship between these two throughout the years. It is also understandable that it has taken me thirty years of groping to reach my present understanding and, at last, to bring it to you.

## You Are More Fortunate Than I Was

No one told me that baldness and diet were related. No one was able to give me rules for retaining, invigorating, and strengthening my hair. But I shall give you those rules that I found so vital to my hair health.

First, let me tell you how it all began. In 1933, when I was a sensitive teen-ager of fourteen, I found myself suffering from a severe case of dandruff. I tried all the common remedies, read the magazine advertisements, listened to the radio commercials, brushed my clothes most carefully when the worthless dandruff "removers" and "preventive shampoos" had failed. Acutely embarrassed and troubled as only an adolescent can be, I went to my family physician. He had helped me and my family out of some pretty tight spots and, since this was the depth of the Depression, he was nice enough to do it without really adequate compensation. I had

learned to rely on him and trust him. But this time I
felt he failed me. He made light of what, even then,
seemed to me an important problem. "Nothing you
can do about it—forget it" was the gist of his advice.
Forget it! When the problem confronted me every day!

For two years I was able to "forget" it by wearing
only gray or tweed jackets. Of course, when I had a date
or went to some relatively "formal" affair, I had to put
on a blue serge suit that showed every speck of dandruff. About this time, the young adolescents started
wearing Oxford gray suits when getting "all dressed
up," which again gave me some respite. But then I was
struck a new blow.

My high school French teacher, Mr. Seybold, called
me "Baldy." I know now that he liked me and was not
trying to be mean or nasty. It was a misguided expression of friendliness and joviality. But think how I, a
sensitive kid looking for an identity, must have felt. I
had been proud of my mop of blond hair—and now it
suddenly became a weakness rather than a source of
strength. Mr. Seybold had noticed a thin spot develop-
ing on the crown and proceeded to tease me about it.
Yet, obviously, neither Mr. Seybold, my family doctor,
nor my concerned parents would have dreamed of connecting my typical teen-age diet of ice cream, soda pop,
and candy with my thinning hair, since this association
was utterly remote from anything they had heard or
studied. What was there for me to do? I changed the
style of my haircut and brushed my hair over the bald
spot, as almost every balding man does. And I contin-

ued to eat sweets in large quantities. And my hair continued to part company with my scalp at an alarming rate for one so young.

### Optimism and Its Limits

So much for my youth. Let's get to your present. A pessimist looks at a pitcher and says, "It's half-empty." An optimist looks at the same pitcher and says, "It's half-full." I have always preferred the optimistic view. But there is a third reaction, that of the scientist, who says, "Let's measure it." My investigations have led me to the conclusion that *I have been able to regrow hair lost within the past five years*. On the average, this should amount to between 15 percent and 25 percent of the hair that has been lost. With persistence and patience in pursuing the program I shall outline, these figures can probably be bettered.

If your scalp is as taut as a drumhead and as shiny as a mirror, it is doubtful that you will be able to help yourself. You must have some viable follicles, some living, even if lazy or sick, hair seeds before you can hope to emulate my success. Here, in outline, is the program that helped me:

### VITAL RULES TO ENCOURAGE THE NUGROW CYCLE

1. Eliminate foods harmful to the scalp and hair.
2. Add to the diet foods rich in germinating substances, vitamins, proteins, and minerals, so that the

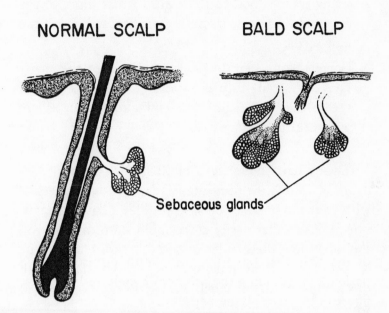

NORMAL SCALP     BALD SCALP

Sebaceous glands

## THE SEBACEOUS GLAND

This illustration shows the sebaceous gland in both the normal and bald scalps. The sebaceous gland produces sebum or oil that lubricates the scalp. An under-productive sebaceous gland can cause a dry scalp while an over-productive gland can cause oily dandruff. Either disorder can be a contributing cause of baldness.

body will produce enzymes and hormones essential to healthy hair growth.

3. Bring more blood to the scalp so that more of the essential nutrients, including oxygen, will reach the hair seeds.

4. Correct your hair hygiene to eliminate the many layers of dead scalp cells and just plain dirt and grease that constitute dandruff and that interfere with healthy hair growth.

If your hair shows signs of ill health—such as dandruff, scalp itch, or thinning—and if you have checked with your physician to be sure you don't have a fungus infection or other easily correctable scalp disease, you should follow these rules as soon as possible. If your scalp becomes tight and shiny, you will be faced with three choices, all of which I shall discuss, and all of which are unpleasant:

1. Accept baldness as a permanent thing and learn to live with it.

2. Wear a wig, toupee, or hairpiece.

3. Have scalp grafted from the hairy fringes that may remain.

# 2

# THE GROWING PROBLEM
# OF BALDNESS

If you were able to make a head count of the more than 200,000,000 persons living in this country, you would find that perhaps 75,000,000 of them are suffering from some hair problem. These problems might be: dry hair, dandruff, excessive hairfall, thinning hair, minor baldness (less than 25 percent loss of hair, or major baldness (greater than 25 percent loss of hair).

Do these statistics sound incredible to you? They are substantiated, among other things, by the wave of new remedies, tonics, and nostrums for hair problems that have flooded the market in the past decades. Turn on your television set and watch the parade of magic potions for rich, glowing hair that fills the screen. You can probably put yourself to sleep counting hair remedies quicker than you can counting sheep.

Another sign of the increase in hair problems is the proliferation of wigs, toupees, and hairpieces. Sometimes I have the eerie feeling, when I go to a party or a meeting, that nearly every man in the room wears a hairpiece. If some magician could turn back the clock and put us back in the days of Washington and Jefferson when powdered wigs were the rage, millions would sigh with relief.

The point I'm making here is that problems connected with hair seem to loom larger every year, and the temptation to sweep those problems under a toupee grows with them. I can understand this feeling. I had an overwhelming urge to try a toupee myself some years ago. Before I formulated the program described in this book, I went to the offices of a toupee manufacturer and looked at his handiwork. Some of it I thought most impressive. I tried one on and submitted to a fitting for a new model designed to do wonderful things for my appearance. But I never went back for a second fitting. Wearing someone else's hair made me feel like a second-class citizen. I just couldn't live with the idea.

This does not mean that I'm ruling out toupees for everyone. Some people simply must have them. I think you'll be able to restore your hair with the kind of diet and care I will recommend in this book, if you're not completely bald. If your scalp is so tight and denuded that nothing grows on it and nothing can grow on it, then a toupee may be your answer. I'll discuss hairpieces in some greater detail as we move along. But most men have *some* hair on their craniums even if it's just a fringe or some fuzz. These men, I am convinced, can be helped to restore their hair through my diet and the rest of my program.

## Don't Blame Hairfall on the Fallout

I began this chapter with some startling figures about the extent of hair problems in America. Have you ever wondered why baldness is increasing?

There is no evidence that it is caused by radioactive fallout, the catchall excuse for unexplained ailments that untrained observers use when they don't know the answers. It is not all heredity. Certainly, heredity does have a role to play in hair problems, but it is not the complete answer. It is not true, as so many people think, that you will be bald because your father was. Neither will you have a full head of hair because your parent was as well-endowed as a Beatle.

If your father had brown eyes, chances are good that you will, too. You may also inherit the shape of his head. But you won't necessarily inherit his lack of hair. The genes don't work that way.

The answer to the startling growth of baldness in the last several decades, I maintain, is the supplanting of a mineral-rich diet of natural, organically grown foods by a menu of diluted, refined, preserved, overcooked foods whose value to the human body has been sharply reduced.

Remember Gresham's law of economics: bad money drives out good. Well, the same thing applies to food.

Bad food (speaking from the standpoint of nutrition, not flavor) has slowly driven out good, healthful food in the kitchens of most of our population. The results have not only affected our general health; they also have helped to make us bald.

## Where Did We Go Wrong?

It all started about a hundred years ago, when the introduction of milling machinery into the manufacture of foodstuffs robbed many foods of their natural body-building values. By turning brown bread into white bread, brown sugar into white sugar, brown rice into white rice, by attacking the native richness of unmilled flour, these machines began slowly to deprive millions of Americans of the mineral values they needed. A long line of denatured foods replaced the organically grown substances that had made our ancestors strong and healthy. The power of many foods to germinate, to help our hair-producing roots perform their work, was curtailed.

How could it be otherwise? When our food was still served to us in its natural state, it still had its vitamins and minerals. They acted as powerful building blocks in producing strong teeth and strong nails. And they helped to produce healthy, luxuriant growths of hair.

Once synthetically fertilized foods took over the dinner table, it was preordained that our hair problems would increase quickly. If you were to study collections of photographs from the time the first camera was developed by Louis Daguerre, you would notice an increasing number of men with balding heads as time went on. I once did just this and I discovered an interesting thing. During the early decades after the 1830s, when daguerreotypes were first created, almost all the men in the photographs had rich, full heads of hair. There were some bald men among them, of course, but their number was small compared to those one notices in the later photographs. In pictures taken after the Civil War, when the synthetically fertilized diets began to take hold, I noticed more and more bald men.

In the century since the Civil War, baldness and hair problems have increased enormously. In the early days of synthetically fertilized foods, man at least continued to consume a substantial percentage of natural foods. Today we are living, most of us, on a diet that is 90 percent demineralized, denatured, and nutritionally deficient.

We eat a steady diet of canned goods, processed meats and cheeses, a host of foods and beverages containing white sugar. Inevitably, it has robbed many of us of the hair we so desperately want to keep.

The tragic thing is that so many people continue to consume these worthless foods, and by doing so risk losing *all* their hair. These are the people I hope to reach in the nick of time, when I come to discuss dietary principles in a later chapter. Since this is a book on hair, I will not at this point go into all the other areas where a natural, healthful diet is also a superior one from the standpoint of general well-being, longevity, and other factors.

The upswing in baldness and hair problems, by the

way, is evident in many countries, not just in America. Wherever the revolution in food-processing methods has denatured the food that people eat, there has been an increase in hair problems. People in European cities buy a great deal of processed food in their own supermarkets these days, and their hair suffers as a direct result. I believe a random sampling of Parisians, Berliners, Londoners, or Romans, compared with an equal sampling of New Yorkers, Chicagoans, or San Franciscans, would reveal almost as high a percentage of persons suffering from dandruff or baldness.

You would not find the same problems, ironically, in more backward areas. In the more primitive parts of the globe—the South Seas, Africa, or Asia—where natural foods are eaten, men and women have full, luxuriant hair growths. The reason is simple: they follow a natural diet that helps to nourish their hair.

Let me give you an even more dramatic illustration of how diet affects the growth and replacement of hair. Take a look at the Hunzukuts of Asia. While baldness is soaring in the rest of the world, it is almost nonexistent among these people.

### Not a Bald Man in Hunza? Pardon Me!
### There Are Exactly Two

The example of the Hunzukuts is heartening to those of us who suffer from hair problems because it shows so convincingly the effects of a healthy diet of natural foods.

Hunza is a tiny, semi-autonomous state located in the Himalayan valley on the northwest frontier of Kashmir. It is nestled between mountain peaks that rise up to 19,000 feet. Understandably, Hunza has remained in almost total isolation from the rest of the world. This is true even though Hunza is only eighteen miles away from where the borders of Russia join with those of Red China and West Pakistan.

Definitely off the beaten path of civilization, Hunza is visited more often by the "Abominable Snowman" than by people from Europe and America. And speaking of the Snowman, if he should ever be caught, we would probably benefit from learning the details of his diet. As you know, the Abominable Snowman is always reported as being exceedingly hairy.

Hunza has a population of 25,000 Hunzukuts—fair-skinned Caucasians of the Moslem faith. They proudly claim as ancestors the soldiers of Alexander the Great. After the campaign against Darius, these soldiers took Persian wives and conveniently lost themselves in the secluded valley of Hunza. Alexander the Great went in the opposite direction, toward civilization, and died at the tragically young age of thirty-three. On the other hand, the typical Hunzukut lives a healthy life until he dies somewhere between the ages of 100 and 120.

## Sex at Ninety! Vigor at 120!

Hunza is a veritable Shangri-la, where the inhabitants lead long, vigorous lives with an enviable freedom from disease. *Even the animals suffer from little or no disease!*

The Hunzukuts are magnificent physical specimens, with amazing powers of endurance. It is not unusual for a man to father children at the age of ninety and to retain his powers of endurance until death comes ten to thirty years later. Hunza must indeed be a man's world, for the men outlive the women by an average of five years; and, because the women spend their days at physical labor, there are no fat women in Hunza. That truly makes it a Shangri-la!

To be sexually potent at ninety. To live past 100. Not one of you reading this book would turn away from such a future! And remember: these powers are the norm for the people of Hunza, not the exception.

There is no great mystery to the secret of Hunza. If you read my first book, *Arthritis and Common Sense*, or if you have heard any of my lectures, you already have learned the answer to the "mystery" of Hunza, as I have analyzed this fascinating riddle.

> Potent sex at ninety.
> A vigorous life to 120.
> *And a full head of hair to 120.*

Is all this something to be desired? Of course it is. But is it impossible to achieve? No, it is *not* impossible. A Hunzukut can father a child at ninety and live with a full head of hair to 120 because of his *diet—a diet of naturally grown products that includes germinating foods.*

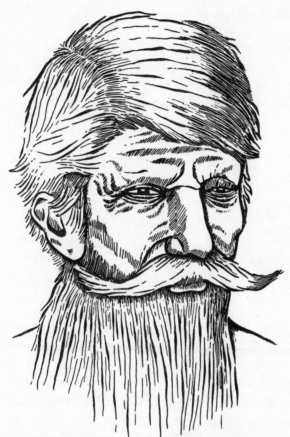

## SEX AT 90—VIGOR AT 120—AND HAIR THE WHOLE WHILE

The typical Hunzukut pictured above lives a healthy life until he dies somewhere between the age of 100 and 120. It is not unusual for a Hunzukut to father a child at the age of 90 and to retain his sexual prowess—and his hair too—until death comes 10 to 30 years later. The text explains what lessons we can learn from the diet of the Hunzukut.

### The Diet of Hunza

To achieve the ideal condition described, the Hunzukut eats the following foods in their natural, unadulterated state: millet, barley, wheat, and buckwheat; turnips, beans, peas, carrots, tomatoes, corn, and potatoes; mutton; cheese, butter, sour milk, and sweet milk.

Then why are there even two bald men in Hunza, and how did they get that way? Two bald—or balding—men live in Hunza. One is the Mir of Hunza (*Mir* means "ruler"), and the other is his brother. The Mir is losing his hair at the crown, and his brother is already three-quarters bald.

Why are the ruler and his brother exceptions to the rule in the paradise of Hunza? Very simple. As princes, they were educated in England. Apparently, they were there long enough to become victims of a "civilized" diet. It would be interesting to learn whether their life span and period of sexual potency were also affected by their extended stay in England as students. Often, when a Hunzukut returns to his valley after spending time in the outside world, he can shed whatever "civilized" ailments he has acquired and return to his naturally healthy condition. The baldness of the rulers, however, suggests that they enjoyed their alien diet and are importing delicacies from the civilized world.

I do not propose that we all migrate to Hunza. But we do have much to learn from the Hunzukuts. *With a proper diet of fresh, organically grown foods, we should be able to approach Hunza's achievements in America.*

## The Happy Polynesians

One of the most fiercely maintained illusions that people have about baldness is that it is caused by exposure to the elements. People get bald, the theory goes, because they go swimming, and the mixture of sun, salt water, and sand just ruins their scalps. Their hair becomes dry and brittle and falls out. I've heard this legend scores of times during my lecture tours around the country.

The next time you visit a public pool or a beach, count the balding men who sit around, wearing hats or berets, afraid to go into the water. They're terrified lest immersion deprive them of their last remaining tufts of hair.

I recall a typical sufferer I met last summer. He was dressed, or perhaps I should say undressed, to the nines: sandals, flamboyant shorts, and the kind of Hawaiian shirt that Harry Truman used to love. And, of course, the inevitable straw hat. Everybody kept urging him to jump into the pool, including a pretty girl he had just met. He gave them all evasive answers.

I took him aside finally and asked him what he was afraid of. He sighed, "I can't go in there. The water would kill my scalp, and the sun's rays would burn it raw. I shouldn't have come down here in the first place. But it's always a temptation when it gets hot. You know how it is."

He was right. He shouldn't have come down. All afternoon he sat by that pool, watching the pretty young things laughing and splashing like happy kids. He longed to jump in, but it was a move he dared not make. The water and sun might make him totally bald, he believed.

But if sun and water create baldness, why is it that the Polynesians, who live in a sun and water world all their lives, have such wonderful hair? How do they retain their magnificent, luxuriant growths?

Fine, you say. But I know men who became bald after several summers of lying around beaches and drenching their hair with salt water. How do you explain that?

I explain it this way. The Polynesians lie around beaches too. They drench their hair with salt water too. But unlike your friends, they don't gorge themselves on refined foods like polished rice, white sugar, and acids of all kinds. They eat a nourishing, protective diet.

Admittedly, constant exposure to the elements will dry the scalp. Sea water must be removed from the scalp or salt will cake on it. But these hazards are also faced daily by the Polynesians. Then why do they seem to be immune to the general tendency toward scalp problems of more civilized peoples? And why, by contrast, do our beach-living friends at home suffer from baldness?

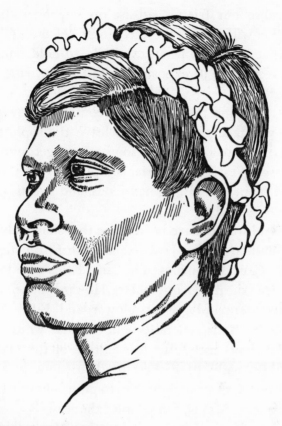

## THE HAPPY POLYNESIAN

If sun and water create baldness, why is it that the Polynesians, who live in a sun and water environment all their lives, retain their magnificent and luxuriant growths of hair? It seems logical to conclude that their diet of nourishing and unrefined foods produces a good growth of hair *in spite of* the effects of salt water, sun, wind, and sand.

Because our friends subsist on improper diets. A good diet will combat the effects of the elements. You've got what it takes, in natural foods, to hold onto your hair, regardless of exposure to salt water, sun, wind, and sand.

You will find much the same contrast wherever you go if you take the trouble to leave the sophisticated modern urban centers. As soon as you get away from our large Western industrial complexes, with their surfeit of canned goods, refined foods, and sweets, the difference is startling.

Several studies have been made that show baldness is less common among Japanese and Chinese males than among Caucasian males. The same holds true for acne and seborrhea. To quote Dr. Howard Behrman, attending dermatologist at Flower and Fifth Avenue Hospitals, "It is generally believed that white people are the most susceptible to baldness of the male pattern type, with the highest predominance in Eastern Mediterranean stock. The Negro groups have less baldness and the Mongolian peoples the least."

In my travels, I have noticed that Mongoloids, Negroids, and certain national subdivisions of the Caucasoids (e.g., Spanish and Portuguese) have more and healthier hair when they stay in their native habitats. In other words, Orientals, Negroes, and Mexicans, to name a few, *show a higher incidence of male pattern baldness at an earlier age when they live a typical American existence. And that typical American existence includes a typical American diet.*

Our society has become the great hair equalizer! If all races continue to eat the American diet of synthetically fertilized, artificially prepared foods, those who predict a totally bald human race for the future may well be right.

In other words, if a Chinese, a Japanese, a Mexican, a Bantu, a Hunzukut, and a Polynesian all decided to live in the United States and shop in our supermarkets, they would be more susceptible to male pattern baldness than if they had remained in their native lands. According to Dr. Behrman, and other experts as well, diet, health, and glandular balance affect hair growth. *And diet affects health and glandular balance.*

Without question, natural selection has determined that peoples living in certain environments will have specific hair patterns and textures. *But, in my opinion, it is diet that is chiefly responsible for most cases of baldness.*

# 3

# DON'T TAKE MY WORD FOR IT—LET'S LISTEN TO WHAT THE SCIENTISTS HAVE TO SAY

At this point, you will be thinking, "Who is Dale Alexander to be giving me advice about health and nutrition? I don't see those magic letters 'M.D.' after his name."

That's a fair comment. I am not a doctor or a scientist and never pretended to be one. But that doesn't prevent me from learning from doctors and scientists, as well as from my own experience.

In addition to Dr. Muller, Dr. Behrman, and other authorities I have quoted and will quote throughout this book, I would now like to bring up some heavy artillery.

A paper of tremendous importance to anyone interested in a healthy head of hair was quietly published in the July, 1967, issue of *Science* magazine (Volume 157). Because of the scholarly character of this publication and its limited circulation, and because of the highly technical language in which the account is written, it made about as much splash in the public's awareness as a pebble dropped into the middle of the Pacific Ocean. Yet here was a description of a scientifically controlled experiment *proving conclusively that if a healthy man is deprived of protein his hair will exhibit severe signs of atrophy and decreased pigmentation, particularly if sugar is substituted for the protein.*

### If You Have a Dictionary, Prepare to Use it Now

Before I quote from this report, prepared by Robert B. Bradfield, Marcelle A. Bailey, and Sheldon Margen, all of the Department of Nutritional Science at the University of California, I must stress that, quite properly, it is presented in technical language. If you find this all a bit abstruse, remember that you challenged me to produce scientific evidence—or, in any event, you probably would have if we were talking face to face—and scientists who write for a technical journal are primarily addressing other scientists. I could not, however, ask you to undertake the strenuous diet proposed in this book without first giving you the scientific foundation on which it is based or, as in this instance, providing recent data that corroborates my previous findings. So pull up your chair, open your dictionary, and read on:

"Eight male subjects," state Bradfield, Bailey, and Margen, "in excellent physical condition aged 24 to 29, were housed in a research ward for more than three months. Physical and biochemical examination showed that they remained in good health throughout the study. The subjects were fed a liquid formula diet three times daily which provided either 75 grams protein per man per day in the form of egg albumen, or else no protein.

"In the latter case Dextri-maltose was substituted isocalorically for the egg albumen. [*My note:* Dextri-maltose is a form of refined sugar obtained from starch.] The diet remained at 2800 calories per man per day throughout the study. . . . At the end of each fifteen-day experimental period approximately 100 hairs were manually plucked from the occipital area of each subject with Tygon-coated needle-holding forceps and examined in a dissecting microscope. Care was taken to use slightly different locations on the scalp in successive samples. . . .

"To avoid bias, both protein-deprived and control subjects were sampled blind at the same time by the same investigator. . . . Consistent morphological changes occurred after the subject was deprived of protein. The hair bulb exhibited severe atrophy and decreased pigmentation. The atrophied bulbs ranged from 0.025 to 0.075 mm. in maximum diameter compared with a range of 0.250 to 0.550 mm. before protein deprivation.

"The morphological changes between the samples taken before and after protein deprivation were consistent in all subjects, although the amount of change varied with the individual. These changes occurred in short-term protein deprivation of normal healthy subjects in the absence of decreases of serum protein, hemoglobin, and hematocrit, and were reversible to some degree when protein was again added to the diet."

### And Now Back to the Plain Old Prose of Plain Old Dale Alexander

From this point on, it is Dale Alexander speaking, and nothing I say should be construed as being the responsibility of the authors of the paper. Nevertheless, if anyone questions whether his diet has any effect on his hair he need only read this report. And if he questions whether the harm caused by an improper diet can be reversed by correcting his eating habits, the answer again seems quite obviously in the affirmative.

During the course of reading—and I hope studying this book—you will be tempted to give it the subtitle of "The Egg and Dale Alexander." Yes, I stress to a fare-thee-well the use of eggs in the diet of anyone interested in improving the health of his hair (along with a drastic reduction in the consumption of sugar). And please note that, in this study, the subjects (except for the ones deprived of protein) were fed their protein in the form of egg albumen.

A point I did not quote from the study but clearly stated in it is that hair breakage, within the follicle, was more frequent in subjects denied egg albumen than in those to whom it was provided. All in all, this little known but truly significant study is the best recent vindication I know of that corroborates my statements regarding the relationship between a sound nutritional program and a healthy head of hair. (Incidentally, to emphasize a point I make elsewhere in this book, anyone whose physician has put him on a low fat and/or low cholesterol diet should consult the physician before adding eggs to his regimen.)

## Meet the Columbuses of Hair Improvement

The ironic thing about the study is that it was not undertaken to determine the effect of diet on the hair but to devise a simple and reliable method of detecting protein-caloric malnutrition. Present diagnostic methods are evidently rather complicated, and simply plucking out a number of hairs and examining them offers a more immediate and inexpensive technique.

This may be another reason why the splash made by this study, which I consider of overwhelming importance to anyone with a hair problem, was so minuscule. Had it been presented as a means of proving that hair can be damaged by a *protein-impoverished sugar-rich* diet and that this damage can be reversed by a protein-rich diet—which is what it indeed does prove—I'm sure the report would not have quietly reposed in the files for more than a year, waiting for Dale Alexander to stumble across it. But no, these three scientists are probably all young men with bushy heads of hair, with completely single-minded devotion to the task they set out to accomplish. Having done so, they presumably turned to other assignments without considering the implications of their discovery. If only one of them had been in the early stages of baldness, the emphasis might have been a bit different!

None of this, of course, has any bearing on the validity of the study. The fact that Columbus was actually seeking a new trade route to India does not detract one iota from the greater significance of his discovery of America. And the fact that Bradfield, Bailey, and Margen were utilizing human hair specifically in their search for a new diagnostic tool in the field of nutrition doesn't alter the fact that they coincidentally proved something of the greatest importance to you, to me, and to everyone else who gets up in the morning and looks at his scalp in the mirror before he even bothers to notice if the rest of his head is still attached to his body.

There is just one additional point I would like to emphasize. Some of you may say, "If lack of protein and too much sugar is injuring my hair, why doesn't it show up in other ways? Why don't my teeth fall out or my arches get flat?" Please turn back and read the opening statement by Bradfield, Bailey, and Margen. They point out that all eight subjects were fed 2,800 calories per man per day throughout the study, which was conducted over a period of more than three months. But four were given 75 grams of protein per man per day in the form of egg albumen and four were deprived of the protein, with sugar (Dextri-maltose) being substituted for it.

The damage to the hair of the latter four was clearly measureable, a damage that fortunately could be reversed by restoring protein to the diet. Yet the three nutritional scientists clearly state that physical and biochemical examination showed that all subjects *remained in good health throughout the study*. This means that hair-root damage can take place without any other physical evidence of ill health when the diet is deficient in proteins, and even when these essential nutrients are replaced by sugar. So don't look for any dramatic warning signals if you are merrily eating your way to baldness. Read this book and ponder its implications.

And now, before we get to a much earlier and more complete study, by Dr. Richard Muller, on nutrition and its effect on hair—the study that first got me started thinking in the right direction, whereas the one discussed in this chapter is primarily a corroboration—I would like to give you more background material on the entire subject. You could easily skip the next chapter, which is about myths and superstitions, and is mostly for fun, but if you've read this book word for word up to this point I hope you will stay with it in sequence the rest of the way. The end justifies the means.

# 4

# MYTHS, SUPERSTITIONS, AND POPULAR BELIEFS

Mankind's fascination with hair seems to be as old as the race itself. Every schoolboy is familiar with the hair that made Samson the most powerful man in the world. Homer referred to the ancient Greeks as "hair-nourishing" men. Archaeologists have found hairpins in Egyptian tombs. And even Aristotle, who was himself losing his hair, expressed interest in the fact that eunuchs, who are not able to grow hair on their chests, do not become bald.

In ancient Greece, it was believed that the application of ravens' eggs to the hair would banish grayness and restore the user's original hair color. The Greeks believed so strongly in this remedy's power to alter color that they kept their mouths filled with oil while using it, lest their teeth be blackened:

The Bible cites a man's hair as the source of his strength, and this idea seems to have been carried down through the centuries. Julius Caesar feared that he was losing his powers along with his hair and attempted desperately to regain his lost hair with massages and tonics, a futile method that millions of men still try today. The Romans, incidentally, forbade anyone to cut his hair while on board ship. Only during a storm was it permissible.

For centuries, the hair of the Mikado of Japan could be cut only while he was asleep, when his soul was presumed to be absent from his body. Otherwise, it was felt that cutting his hair might injure his soul.

In Tyrolia, witches were said to create hail and thunderstorms with shed hair, while in medieval England the life span of the individual was estimated by the hair on his forehead. If his hair grew low on the forehead and retreated above the temples, it was said a long life was indicated.

## Remedies

History has also handed down some bizarre cures for baldness. Long before Cleopatra sailed the Nile, men were searching for ways to stop falling hair.

The earliest remedy on record comes from the Ebers Papyrus, thought to have been written in Egypt around 1550 B.C. The remedy was a mixture of fats from the ibex, lion, crocodile, serpent, goose, and hippopotamus. Along with this, the balding sufferer was advised to take

burned prickles of a hedgehog immersed in oil, fingernail scrapings, and a potpourri of honey, alabaster, and
red ocher, all with the proper incantations.

There are no records showing whether this prescrip-
tion worked or not, and I haven't tried it myself since
I don't own an ibex, but we do know that wigs were
popular in ancient Egypt.

Hand in hand with the old wives' remedies for hair
loss have been the taunts and jests hurled at its victims.
The bald have been laughed at by the man in the street
and by those in seats of power. Indeed, there were a
number of kings who retained bald jesters, the better
to tease them. The gibes have continued through the
centuries and some of them have come from men who
should have known better.

Samuel Johnson, as late as the eighteenth century,
dogmatically stated that bald men are stupid. "The
cause of baldness in man," harrumphed the great lexi-
cographer, "is dryness of the brain, and its shrinking
from the skull."

## Popular Myths About Baldness

Let's face it. Taunts directed at bald men, like gibes
about fat men, will never end nor will the making of
many myths about baldness ever come to an end. During many years of lecturing throughout this country
and abroad, I have heard some mighty odd notions. I
also learned that the average man knows next to
nothing about hair loss. Here are a few of the questions

I posed to people and some of the answers I got. Mind you, most of these people were intelligent men and women who showed a good deal of common sense in talking on other subjects.

QUESTION: Why do you think men get bald?
ANSWERS: Diseases, heredity, worry, smoking, neglect, wearing of tight hats, not wearing hats at all, the tensions of our society, too much sex, too much sun and wind and water, washing the hair too often, not washing it often enough.
QUESTION: What foods do you think are good for the hair?
ANSWERS: Beer, fish, oranges, proteins.
QUESTION: What causes dandruff?
ANSWERS: Dry scalp, failure to wash, failure to use hair tonics, living in a dry atmosphere, drinking highly chlorinated water, eating foods containing calcium, eating fried foods.

I found that many people have firm convictions about the effect of food on hair, but they cannot explain the physiological reactions involved. And they have no notion whatsoever about cause and effect when it comes to diet and hair. A number of college students told me, for instance, that they thought drinking frozen orange juice would cause a person's hair to turn gray. A number of others attributed grayness to the consumption of grapefruit juice and pink lemonade. These ideas are, of course, arrant nonsense.

The idea that heredity is a basic cause of baldness has validity. Heredity *is* a factor. But because the father is bald it does not necessarily mean his son will be bald. It is true that, like the shape of a man's chin, his teeth, the color of his eyes, a man's hair growth is in part pre-ordained by his genes. But the offspring of a father with big ears do not all have large ears, and children of a bald father do not all suffer from baldness.

There is a difference between *inheriting* a character-istic and *expressing* that inheritance. For example, it is known that most cases of diabetes are an *expression* of an *inherited tendency* toward diabetes. However, in many cases, if a fat diabetic loses weight, his diabetes may become latent and not express itself for decades. It may take some stress, such as an operation, a severe ill-ness, a physical or mental shock, or a dietary indiscre-tion to make the diabetes reappear. Similarly, one may inherit a *tendency* toward baldness, but it may not *express* itself as a bald spot unless some untoward event occurs. And too much sun, heat, or, above all, dietary indiscretion may be the stressful event that allows an inherited tendency to dandruff to become manifest.

I am convinced that your rate of hair growth, or the rate of loss of your hair, is decided in large part by what you eat or fail to eat. If a faulty diet can affect hard organs like teeth and bones, it can assuredly affect the hair. Hair is as susceptible to substances carried in the bloodstream as are the teeth and bones.

It appalls me to hear a man say, "My father was bald, so I'm going to be bald. Why should I bother to make the effort to save hair that is bound to go?" This defeatist attitude is based upon a superficial understanding of heredity and a complete *lack* of understanding of the manifold factors that affect hair growth.

Another myth connected with baldness is that bald men are sexier. (As a man whose hair is relatively thin, I hate to explode this belief.) It probably arose because the general public knows that there is some connection between the male sex hormone, testosterone, male baldness, and abundant body hair. However, sexiness depends not only on the presence of the male sex hormone but also upon psychological adjustment. A bald man with a hairy body and with plenty of male hormone who is not sure of his virility will not be sexy; conversely, cases have been reported of postpubertal male castrates who can still get erections and enjoy sexual intercourse, although the testes that manufacture testosterone have been removed. If it were true that bald men are the sexiest, men would be seeking hair *removers* rather than hair *restorers*.

Part of this same myth is the belief that too much sexual activity will cause a man to lose his hair. How much is "too much"? Havelock Ellis describes the case of a couple who had intercourse at least once every night for decades. Ellis doesn't mention whether the husband was bald.

My informants across the country also were quick to

blame service in the armed forces for the loss of their hair. They ascribed it variously to the heavy, tight hats, to dirt and the inability to keep clean, to the too-frequent showers they were forced to take, to heavily chlorinated water, or to the nervous tension generated by the insecurities of military life. It is my belief that the military diet, running heavily to grease and fried foods, supplemented at the PX by large quantities of ice cream, candy, and pop, is more responsible for this hair loss. It is common, PX managers have told me, for a man to buy a full box of a dozen candy bars, to consume it before nightfall, and to return the next day for another box. It is true that young men are often "nervous in the service." Some try to "sweeten" their lives with ice cream and candy, both of which contain refined sugar. This sugar, I believe, is a more vital cause of baldness than any other factor.

Some people think that daily showers are not harmful *if* one uses a soapless shampoo. How many young men in the service—or out of it, for that matter—know enough to buy a soapless shampoo rather than use any piece of soap that lathers?

Lastly, I am convinced that *no medicament rubbed into the scalp* and *no medication taken by mouth* ever caused a single new hair to grow. Many of these quack remedies are on the market and are being touted daily over television. People spend millions of dollars and millions of hours of time buying these nostrums and belaboring their scalps. The most they accomplish is to remove some of the dandruff temporarily and to increase the local blood circulation for even less time. There is no lasting benefit.

On the other hand, thirty years of self-observation has convinced me that, *with a constructive program based primarily on diet, I stopped my hair loss and grew new hair in significant quantity and on schedule.* Forget all the myths and old wives' tales you have ever heard. Let's get down to cause and effect.

# 5

# THE STRUCTURE AND
# GROWTH OF YOUR HAIR

"Man is a bizarre mammal; reflect upon the absurdity of an animal with a practically naked skin, with rich tufts of hair growing here and there over its body. We are at a loss to find a function for these strange tussocks of hairs. I propose that this hair is an ornament as is the mane of the lion and some Old World monkeys." So said Montagna, in the *Archives of Dermatology*, July, 1963. Although the function of human hair eludes us, the anatomy of the hair has been well described. I shall acquaint you with this structure so that you will be knowledgeable when I refer to the hair papilla, the hair follicle, and other terms in subsequent chapters.

I realize that much of this material is difficult reading, but I'm not worried that anyone who is partially bald will refuse to devote a few hours of concentration to this book. I know only too well from my own experience that anyone in our special "class" will wade through a library, let alone a book, if he is convinced it will help him graduate from that class.

Incidentally, if I sound like a *herr Doktor* professor, or "hair doctor" if you prefer, it is only because I have interviewed many specialists and studied many textbooks in the course of my researches on the subject. I make no claim to a medical degree or professional standing. It's just that I have digested a great deal of pertinent information and am feeding it back to you, in relatively convenient form, so that you will know what you are doing in your quest and why you are doing it. As I said before, the subject is important enough to justify a bit of extra effort on the part of both of us.

## The Scalp

We start with the scalp. This is the covering of the upper part of the head from the skin to the bone. From the outside in, the scalp consists of: the skin; the subcutaneous tissue, made of fat and fibrous tissue; the epicranium, which is formed by the two fleshy bellies of the occipitofrontalis muscle and the flattened tendon between them; then a layer of thin fibrous tissue called areolar tissue, which allows for movement of the upper scalp. It was this layer that made it easy for the American Indians and the ancient Scythians to scalp their foes. The deepest layer is the pericranium, which is really the covering of the skull bone.

Some people have a talent for contracting the two bellies of the occipitofrontalis muscle alternately, thus producing a wagging movement in their scalps. They are usually proud of this ability, though why it should be a matter for human pride I don't know, since monkeys can do it better. Distributed in the subcutaneous tissue are tortuous arteries that form a connecting network across the midline with their fellows of the opposite side, an unusual arrangement in the body. These arteries, when cut, bleed freely because their mouths are held open by the dense fibrous tissue in which they lie.

There are also veins, lymphatic vessels, and nerves. Judging from the copious blood supply, the scalp would seem to be an important organ for the body and is served accordingly.

## Hair Follicles

The scalp is more richly supplied with hair follicles than any other portion of the skin. A hair follicle is a small pocket pushing into the skin from the surface, at the bottom of which is a cluster of cells, called the matrix, from which the hair grows. This matrix, in the human scalp, will produce on the average 0.35 millimeter—a little more than 1/100 of an inch—of hair per day. The energy required of the body's metabolism to produce this amount of hair is extremely large compared with that required to produce other bodily tissues. If this requirement is not met by the products brought to the follicle in the bloodstream, the hair will not grow, or, if it does, it will not be very healthy.

Closely associated with the hair is a small sebaceous gland that produces an oil called sebum. Overproduction of sebum is a disease condition called seborrhea, which is often associated with dandruff. We will discuss seborrhea and dandruff at greater length in a later chapter.

The hair follicle is lined with the upper layers of the skin, which are continuous with the surface of the scalp. The follicle is widest at its base, which is called the bulb. Inside the bulb is a hole filled with loose connective tissue, the latter called the dermal papilla.

The hair stands in the center of the follicle with its root extending down to the bulb. A hair may be divided into an inner medulla and a much thicker outer cortex, surrounded by sheaths and membranes. It is, microscopically, much more complex than it seems to the naked eye; but a detailed discussion of the microscopic anatomy is not necessary for our purpose.

When a follicle stops producing a hair, whatever the reason, it shrivels up; and the bulb largely degenerates. This is called the telogen, or resting phase. The growing follicle is called the anagen. The transition phase between the two is referred to as the catagen. At the base of the resting follicle the hair forms a club. Below the base of the club hair is a basal epithelial peg which, with the lower part of the sheath, forms the hair germ,

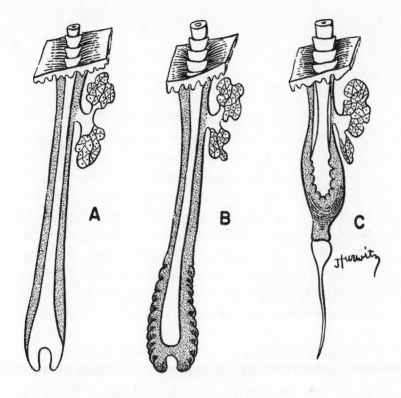

## CROSS SECTION OF THE HAIR FOLLICLE

The three stages of development of the Hair Follicle are illustrated in this cross section. They are:

A. The *Anagen* or growing follicle.
B. The *Catagen* or transition stage.
C. The *Telogen* or resting stage. At this point the follicle shrivels up and the bulb degenerates.

or matrix, from which the next generation of hairs develops.

## Pigmentation and Texture

Considerably above the bulb but still below the surface of the skin, the cells lose their structure and flow together; we call this process keratinization. Above the matrix, the hair becomes pigmented, the pigment-producing cells, or melanocytes, living in the upper bulb. Black and brown pigments are very similar chemically; yellow pigment is different and probably akin to the pigment of red hair. Little is known, unfortunately, about the inheritance of hair color in man. But with tints and dyes so readily available, today's humans—at least the female of the species—don't let that worry them.

What we think of as the hair is really the pigmented, keratinized shaft that extends from just under the skin to the tip, be it crew-cut or Beatle-banged. From the preceding short discussion of hair origin and growth, it is easy to understand that the quality of the hair cannot possibly depend upon what you smear upon it, but must derive from the health of the hair matrix and scalp. And that, in turn, depends upon the circulation and quality of the blood brought to it.

When a hair follicle reaches the end of its cycle of growth, a club hair is formed above the bulb; and the bulb is almost entirely destroyed, leaving the follicle much shorter. When growth starts again in that follicle,

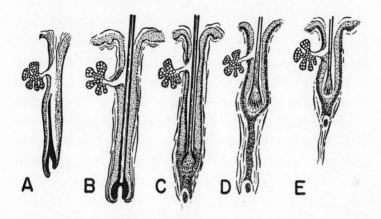

## THE GROWTH CYCLE OF A HAIR

Five stages in the growth of a hair are depicted here, in cross section, portraying the growth cycle up to the point of formation of a club hair.

The stages are:

*A.* New Hair
*B.* Growing Hair
*C.* Presumptive Club Hair
*D.* Emergent Club Hair
*E.* Mature Club Hair

When a hair follicle reaches the end of its cycle of growth (the *Telogen* phase) a club hair is formed above the bulb. (The bulb is then almost entirely destroyed.) Below this club hair is a basal epithelial peg. When NuGrowth starts again, this peg, along with the lower part of the sheath, forms the matrix, or hair germ, which then rebuilds the bulb from which the next generation of hair develops.

the hair germ rebuilds a bulb, which then sprouts a hair.

In cross section, straight hair is round and curly hair is oval or flattened. Diameters of one strand of hair range from 1/1,500 to 1/140 of an inch. In general, flaxen hair is the finest and black the coarsest. The scalp contains about 120,000 hairs, or 1,000 hairs to the square inch. Blonds have the most, averaging about 140,000 hairs, while redheads have the least—about 90,000. Women generally have more hairs per inch than men. Hairs live, on the average, two to six years, though in some individuals they may live much longer.

## A Capsule Commentary on Gray Hair

The graying of hair results from the aging of the pigment cells, or melanocytes. As early as 1921, Bloch, working in Germany, showed that in older persons with gray hair there was markedly diminished melanin formation in the hair bulbs. In elderly subjects with snowy-white hair, he found no melanin at all. Lately, this condition has been shown to be due to the gradual loss of activity of an enzyme called tyrosinase in the hair bulb melanocytes. In total albinos, no tyrosinase activity can be detected in the hair follicles. This peculiarity is controlled by an inherited gene. Pigmentary deficiencies may also be found in a localized area, such as one white forelock. While the total albino *does* have melanocytes, these are unpigmented. The white forelock is also due to lack of tyrosinase activity.

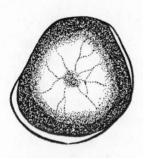

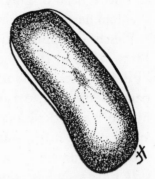

## Straight hair          ## Curly hair

## STRAIGHT vs. CURLY

What makes a hair decide to lead a crooked life or go straight?
Basically, it is the shape of the hair. As shown here in cross section,
straight hair is normally round in shape and curly hair is oval.
Artificial restraint, teasing, and other forms of torture can make
straight hair temporarily curly and vice versa, but it will always
try to regain its natur·l condition.

A head of gray hair usually turns out, on closer inspection, to be a mixture of normally colored hairs, white hairs, and gray hairs. It is most unusual to have an entire head of gray hair, although many of the individual hairs may actually be gray.

Flesch, in a publication of the University of Chicago Press, wrote in 1954 that hair growth may be impaired by deficiencies of vitamin A, riboflavin, biotin, inositol, pantothenic acid, pyridoxine, and vitamin E. Most of his work was done on animals and is not necessarily applicable to man, but similar studies were done directly on humans. A great deal of work with humans still remains to be done before we know the entire story.

Lanczos, writing in 1941, found that vitamin B, *taken over a long period,* restored human hair pigmentation. A British investigator, Hughes, demonstrated in 1946 that a deficiency of the B vitamins known as riboflavin and pantothenic acid not only caused hair depigmentation in Negro children, but also caused their hair to grow straight. It has been suggested that patients deficient in pantothenic acid cannot utilize copper. In sheep, a deficiency of copper causes sheep to produce straight wool that is deficient in pigment.

We must conclude that, while much more needs to be learned about hair growth, vitamin and mineral deficiencies have been detected in the abnormal growth of hair in animals and in man. Knowledge in this field is still in its infancy, but it seems obvious that further study will prove the importance of diet.

# 6

## BALDNESS: WHAT IS IT?

Baldness is a subdivision of what the skin specialists refer to as hypotrichosis, meaning absence or abnormal sparseness of hair. If this hypotrichosis occurs on the scalp, it is termed baldness. There are many classifications of hypotrichosis. These are the main ones:

1. *Primary hypotrichosis,* where the loss of hair is due to some pathological condition in the hair follicle, bulb, or shaft.
2. *Secondary hypotrichosis,* where the loss of hair is secondary to some type of disease that is not primarily located in the hair but involves hair loss as one of its symptoms. Examples of this type of hair loss, which do not concern us in this book, are syphilis, fungus diseases of the skin, certain skin diseases that result in a drying up or atrophy of the skin, and certain skin infections.

67

The ordinary type of baldness we see all about us is considered a form of primary hypotrichosis and is called *alopecia prematura* or *alopecia seborrheica*. The word "alopecia" comes from the Greek word *alope,* meaning "fox." My predecessors in baldness research fancied that the bald pate resembled that of a fox suffering from mange, so they called baldness "alopecia." More appropriate would have been a Greek word for billiard ball, but the ancient Greeks didn't play billiards. *Alopecia prematura* is a common condition occurring almost exclusively in men. In the textbook *Dermatology: Essentials of Diagnosis and Treatment* by two of America's leading skin specialists, Sulzberger and Wolff, it is stated that "the affliction is unquestionably associated with hereditary and familial tendencies related to those leading to acne vulgaris and seborrhea." They also say: "It is usual to find scaly seborrhea (dandruff) and, later, an oily scalp as an early manifestation of the process. These may constitute an *additional* factor in the early loss of hair . . . but are not *obligatory* concomitants or proved causes." (The italicizing of the word "additional" is mine.) They conclude the paragraph with: "Many persons with severe dandruff and oily scalp never become bald, while in some persons with early pronounced baldness there is no evidence of any preceding dandruff or oiliness of the scalp." And the next paragraph I find *most* significant: "Although elimination of the coexisting seborrhea and stimulation of the scalp may retard hair loss, the ultimate progression is *almost* unaltered by treatment." To me, in the light of my investigations into my own hair problem, this adds up to the following:

1. Conventional treatment is unavailing.
2. An important factor is left uninvestigated in the professors' discussion of the therapy of baldness. (This is not intended as a reflection on two of the nation's leading dermatologists; the scientists who preceded Newton can hardly be "blamed" for failing to make the discoveries that he subsequently hit upon.)
3. That factor is diet, *diet,* and, above all, DIET.

Another type of rather common alopecia is *alopecia areata.* This disease is usually found only in the hair or beard but at times affects all the hairy areas of the body. If all the hair of the body disappears, the condition is termed *alopecia universalis;* if it involves the entire scalp, but not the rest of the body, it is called *alopecia totalis.* The cause of *alopecia areata* is at present unknown, although many of the reported cases occurred after sudden psychological shocks. In fact, many cases have been reported in which a person has a psychic trauma one day and wakes up the next morning to find a group of hairs lying on the pillow and a bald patch on his scalp where hair had been growing the night before.

Occasionally, the appearance of the bald patch is heralded by slight redness and itching, or stinging, or a severe headache. It differs from *alopecia prematura* in that it strikes both sexes equally and may appear at

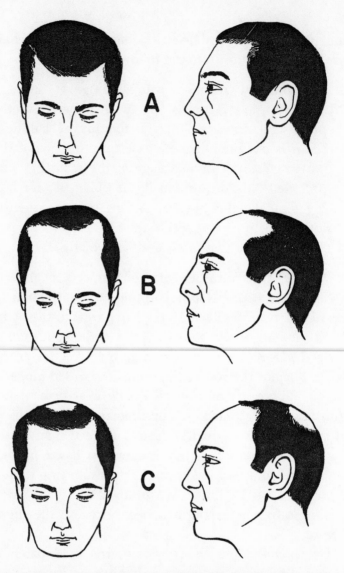

**VARIOUS STAGES OF MALE PATTERN BALDNESS**

Male Pattern Baldness follows a definite progression, as explained above, and is found typically in males or in females with a glandular condition in which too much male hormone is produced. It differs

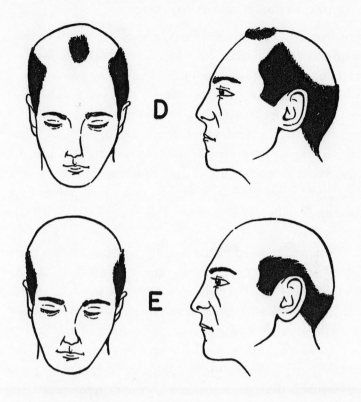

from alopecia (baldness) of other types which have other patterns or no pattern at all.

- **A.** Normal hair growth.
- **B.** The receding hairline. Usually the first manifestation of Male Pattern Baldness is the recession of the hairline along the temporal area.
- **C.** The appearance of loss at the crown. As the hairline moves back, the loss starts at the crown and moves forward.
- **D.** The lamentable meeting of the two areas of defoliation. At this stage only a small "island" of hair remains in the frontal area, as the bald spot at the crown has moved to both front and rear.
- **E.** "Fait Accompli!" The pattern, so familiar to all of us, has run its course. In males the hair loss usually stops here. Hence the term "Male Pattern Baldness."

any age. If it occurs after forty, and if it goes on to total baldness or universal hair loss, the prognosis for full recovery is much less favorable than in the patchy cases, which usually recover in one to two years. The first hairs to reappear are usually very fine, like that on a newborn baby, and are often gray or white. They usually return to their normal color eventually, but not always. It is paradoxical that fashionable ladies who highlight their hair with one or two white patches are unconsciously imitating one of the stages of this disease of the hair.

Now we come to forms of alopecia that can be diagnosed and treated only by a trained medical doctor. In fact, if your family doctor, whether a general practitioner or family internist, suspects any of these diseases, he will usually send you to a dermatologist to confirm his suspicions and suggest the proper treatment. These much more rare forms of baldness include *alopecia syphilitica* due to secondary (generalized) syphilis; alopecia due to tertiary (gummatous) syphilis; alopecia due to superficial noninflammatory fungi, such as *Microsporon audouini* or *Trichophyton violaceum;* alopecias that accompany such systemic diseases as *lupus erythematosus;* and alopecias following X-ray or radium treatment, local infections like boils and carbuncles, or poisons such as arsenic in large doses. All these conditions need skilled care, and no attempt should be made to treat them at home with diet or any other remedy not prescribed by your physician.

## Her Crowning Glory—Is She Losing Her Throne?

In 1960, Drs. Sulzberger, Witten, and Kopf became alarmed by what seemed to be a sharp increase in diffuse hair loss in females. They queried 106 of the leading dermatologists of North America and recorded the answers to their questionnaires in the American Medical Association's *Archives of Dermatology* for April, 1960. Over half of the skin specialists confirmed that they had observed increases in hair loss in females in recent years. Dermatologists from Italy and France have reported similar findings. While a few female patients have noticed sudden loss of large amounts of hair, some have felt that it was lost in spurts, with periods of increased or decreased hair-loss activity. But in most patients, the loss of hair has been insidious, slow but steady. After months or years, it is obvious that a formerly luxuriant growth has become sparse.

Since women usually wear their hair longer than men, it is easier for them to conceal the damage; but the psychological trauma is perhaps even greater, since girls are brought up to glory in their tresses and consider them one of their chief sexual attractions and adornments. The millions of dollars and millions of hours spent annually at hairdressers' testify to the major importance of hair to women in our culture. And not only in *our* culture. Throughout the world, from the most primitive Australian pigmy tribe through the harems of Saudi Arabia to the most soignée Parisian demimondaine, the hair is turned, twisted, pomaded, oiled, perfumed, lacquered, and adorned until any resemblance to the original tresses is purely accidental. Presumably, all this effort produces some desired effect on the male; otherwise intelligent women would not have pursued this time- and energy-consuming art for all these millennia.

To get back to Sulzberger *et al.*, they mention that the hair shafts of their women patients became thin or wiry and lost their pliancy or luster. The process may affect the entire scalp but usually involves only the dome or sides toward the front. Female baldness does not usually progress to the extreme degree seen in men. Only a few patients seem to have regrown their hair after a number of months or years. No cause for this condition has been found as yet, and no specific treatment.

## Traction Baldness

Dr. H. V. Morgan, of the University of Khartoum in the Sudan, has described, in the *British Medical Journal* for July, 1960, a form of baldness found in tribal women of the northern Sudan who plait their hair into many small plaits, sometimes numbering 120 or more. They usually incorporate black silk threads in these plaits and may add as much as sixteen ounces of thread. This plaiting is all done near the middle of the scalp and leads to a denuded area in the midline where the plaits pull on the scalp.

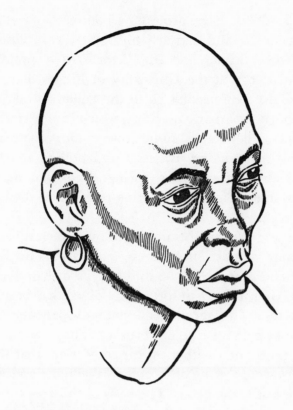

## TOO MUCH PONY TAIL?

The tribal woman of Northern Sudan, pictured above, pulls her hair into many small plaits, sometimes numbering 120 or more. This may lead to what is known as traction baldness. While hair loss in women does not usually progress to the extreme degree seen in men, 106 dermatologists, queried by Drs. Sulzberger, Witten, and Kopf in 1960, agree that the diffuse types of hair loss in women from 20 to 40 years of age is on the upswing. Traction baldness seems to be one of the reasons for this upswing. The above is an example of the most extreme results of traction baldness.

Dr. Rudolph Baer, professor of dermatology at the renowned Skin and Cancer Unit of New York University Medical School, and Dr. Victor Witten, professor of dermatology at the University of Miami, have remarked that one needn't go to the Sudan to find evidence of such barbaric practices, which cause "traction alopecia." They state: "In our own country, hair fashions call for winding, twisting, and pulling the hair around clips, pins, rollers, springs, and even barbed devices, in each instance exerting traction on the hairs of the scalp."

Baer and Witten also implicate the ponytail hairdo as a cause of traction baldness, and agree with Sulzberger and others that the diffuse type of hair loss in women from twenty to forty years of age has been on the increase. They recommend that their patients avoid the use of nylon bristle hairbrushes. They also recommend, apparently without great conviction, that their patients avoid the use of "soapless" shampoos and stick to pure castile shampoos. The basis of this reasoning is that most, *but not all*, of these female patients had been using soapless shampoos before they became bald. I do not agree with this reasoning. Here's why: Sulzberger, Witten, and Kopf remark, "Many of these patients note increased oily seborrhea of the scalp in association with hair loss." When oily seborrhea occurs in the male, these same authorities are apt to recommend a soapless shampoo.

Even the most eminent dermatologists would admit

that their science is still a young one. It is still based, to a large extent, on trial and error, on empiricism, on tradition. Baldness is just one of the many riddles as yet unanswered by dermatologists.

## Where Does That Leave Us?

To summarize what is known for sure about female baldness, we may state that a relatively few cases are caused by hair styles pulling on the scalp. A few others are due to the overproduction of male hormone in the female due to a pathological lesion in the ovaries, the adrenal glands, or the pituitary. But the majority of cases are of unknown origin.

As far as I am concerned, I feel that, just as too little attention has been paid to diet in *alopecia seborrheica* in the male, so too the question of diet in female alopecia has been neglected. Can the change from fresh to canned and frozen vegetables and meats in our diet, as well as the increasing vogue for denatured foods and the failure to consume fresh sprouting or germinating foods (except for sprouting potatoes, which are quite harmful), be the factor that these two types of alopecia have in common?

Perhaps male hormone accounts for the *pattern* of baldness but not for its occurrence. Perhaps heredity determines in whom baldness is *apt* to occur but does not foreordain that it actually takes place. Perhaps the correct diet will so strengthen the hair root that it can

better withstand the effects of male hormone, of heredity, of the 101 factors of everyday living, so many of
which are deleterious to the hair. In my case, carefully
chosen food has, in my own experience, not only
stopped my hair from falling but has helped me regrow
most of the hair I lost in the past five years.

# 7

# DANDRUFF, SEBORRHEA, AND HAIR LOSS

Dandruff refers to the shed scales of the surface of the scalp, which either become entangled in the hair or fall on a dark surface and so become noticeable. It is normal for every scalp to have some dandruff. Excessive amounts may be due to a condition called seborrhea. Seborrheic dermatitis of the scalp is a chronic inflammatory disease of the skin, one which begins in the scalp and later may spread to the eyebrows, eyelids, ears, the region where the nose joins the cheek, the edges of the lips, over the breast bone, the armpits, and several other areas. The disease is characterized by dry or moist or greasy scales and sometimes by pinkness and crusted patches, as well as by some itching. The disease may wax or wane or, to use more scientific language, show exacerbations and remissions.

As far as you and I are concerned, it is only seborrhea of the scalp that interests us. The least severe phase is a dry, branny, flaky scaling referred to as *pityriasis sicca*. These two words are favorites of the dermatologists, who seem to find it easier to describe a condition in ancient Greek or Latin than in modern English. In this case, they combined the Greek word for "bran" with the Latin word for "dry," making a curiously euphonious hodgepodge.

*Pityriasis sicca* begins as a dry peeling in small patches, spreading rapidly to involve the entire scalp surface with a profuse coating of fine powdery scales. The next stage is *pityriasis steatoides*. Here, at least, the dermatologists used only Greek, *steatoides* meaning "fatlike" in that ancient language. It refers to an oily type of dandruff, at times accompanied by redness and perhaps by an accumulation of thick crusts.

Andrews and Domonkos, both respected consultants in skin diseases at New York's Columbia Presbyterian Medical Center, say in their textbook *Diseases of the Skin*: "There is a tendency for the hair in the affected areas to fall out, characteristically beginning on the vertex and frontal regions and progressively receding. It is commonly associated with premature baldness in men." More severe stages manifest greasy scaling patches or thick, scaling eruptions that may ooze and become thickly crusted. In the most severe cases, the entire scalp may be covered by a malodorous, dirty crust. In infancy, this is known as cradle cap.

Andrews and Domonkos continue: "The etiology of seborrheic dermatitis is undetermined. . . . Many patients with the disease have low basal metabolic rates, and eat excessively of *sweets, starches, or fats.*" They neglect to define *what kind* of sweets, starches, and, especially, fats. I shall attempt to remedy that neglect. They do mention that alcoholic drinks, chocolate, or sweets are harmful, and that a deficiency of vitamin B is found in some cases. Among the treatments they recommend as helpful are vitamin B complex and $B_{12}$, riboflavin, and nicotinamide. They stress the importance of scalp cleanliness.

The expert called upon to discuss seborrhea for the *Encyclopaedia Britannica* states that on the head, where it is commonly seen, seborrhea may interfere with the nutrition of the hair and cause partial baldness. And Flesch and his colleagues report the temporary loss of hair, with disappearance of most of the hairs and their follicles, when human sebum and three of its components, squalene, oleic, and linoleic acids, were applied *only once* to the skin of laboratory animals. The hair loss began ten to twelve days after the application; similar results could not be produced in a control series with the use of mineral oil, lanolin, or stearic acid.

While the presence of dandruff or of seborrhea does not *necessarily* mean that the hair will be lost, it is about the only warning signal we have. I feel that it is safer to heed this warning and attempt to save one's hair, rather than to wait to see whether one belongs to the category of hairless seborrheic or that of hairy seborrheic. It may be true that less than 50 percent of seborrheics lose hair; but it is also true that for each individual who becomes bald, he is 100 percent his own statistic!

## You and Your Sebaceous Glands

Whatever the factors that cause the scalp to age— and I, as you know by now, have my own ideas about these factors—they obviously affect the hair follicles much more intensely than they affect the sebaceous and sweat glands. It is common knowledge to the learned investigators of the skin that, as Ellis of Brown University and others have shown, the sebaceous glands in the infant scalp are small. In young men, they are considerably larger. In the aged, nonbalding scalp, the sebaceous glands are still larger and more complex. And finally, in bald scalps, the sebaceous glands are very large and very complex. In fact, Ellis says that they become the most conspicuous organs in the scalp.

Why is it that the hair follicles gradually wither, while the other organs of the scalp show ever-increasing luxuriant growth? No one knows for sure, but I am convinced that improper diet starves and poisons the follicles and that this felony is compounded, so to speak, because the same improper diet simultaneously overnourishes the oil glands.

Many years ago, when scientific investigation of the

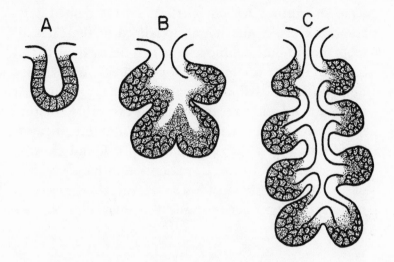

## DEVELOPMENT OF THE SEBACEOUS GLANDS

The Sebaceous Glands are a group of glands, surrounding the hair follicles, which secrete oily matter, called sebum, for the lubrication of hair and skin in both animals and man. The degree of secretion of these glands can greatly affect the health of the hair. The illustration above depicts the relative appearance of these glands at various steps of human development.

*A.* Sebaceous Glands at infancy.

*B.* Normal adult growth where the secretion of sebum is in good balance: neither too little nor too much.

*C.* Baldness. Where baldness exists, the sebaceous glands are very large and very complex. In fact, they become the most conspicuous organs in the scalp. Improper diet may cause these glands to produce excessive amounts of sebum, which in turn can contribute to baldness.

scalp was just beginning, a fungus was found on the scalp of persons with seborrhea. It was named *pityrosporum ovale*, and it was acclaimed as the cause of seborrhea and of baldness. It is still being depicted in some television commercials for dandruff "cures." But now we know that this is a harmless organism that thrives on oil and likes to live in the favorable environment provided by a greasy scalp. Later investigators showed that *pityrosporum ovale* may be found growing profusely on the scalps of patients who have *no* signs of seborrhea. So we must bid an unregretful farewell to notions of *pityrosporum ovale* as a cause of seborrhea or baldness.

## How to Get Rid of Seborrhea of the Scalp

Let us consider first what a typical dermatological textbook says about the treatment of seborrhea of the scalp, and then let us see if my own nonprofessional recommendations do not seem to strike a more hopeful note.

Andrews and Domonkos suggest shampooing once weekly and perhaps twice a week if the scalp is excessively oily. For very oily scalps, they recommend tincture of green soap or a 5 percent solution of sodium lauryl sulfate, which is a "spreading agent." They state that selenium sulfide shampoo gives excellent results but tends to make the hair oily if used too frequently.

I may add that, in some susceptible persons, it may also thin the hair. They state that the benefits of ultraviolet radiation are widely recognized.

They also suggest Grenz ray therapy, which is a form of superficial X-ray exposure. Unless the seborrhea is so marked as to be disabling, I would certainly hesitate to recommend, on the basis of the experts I have consulted, radioactive therapy of any kind. There are too many possible harmful effects.

In addition to the vitamins mentioned earlier, they also suggest crude liver extract injections. I feel that it has never been shown that crude liver extract contains any active ingredient beyond vitamin $B_{12}$. If you *like* injections, vitamin $B_{12}$ hurts a lot less than crude liver and, due to the miracles of modern mass production, doesn't cost any more.

They also feel that thyroid extract is indicated. I have discussed this with an endocrinologist friend. He tells me that, unless the patient is definitely hypothyroid, thyroid extract will do him no good. He also points out that in a patient who is not hypoglandular, the administration of any glandular substance, thyroid or any other, suppresses the function of the pituitary gland so that no more of that particular substance is produced by the target gland, in this case the thyroid. Then the patient ends up with the same amount of thyroid in his body that he would have had if the thyroid extract had not been given.

To shorten a story that threatens to become too technical—even though I warned you I would have to tax your powers of concentration—let me sum it up by saying that thyroid extract is of value if, and only if, the patient does not have enough thyroid hormone of his own. Then it is indicated for the hypothyroidism, not for the seborrhea specifically.

In severely and acutely inflamed cases, the dermatologists recommended antibiotics, and cortisone-like medication or ACTH, the pituitary hormone that stimulates the adrenal gland to produce in the body cortisone-like products of its own. There can be no quarrel with a physician administering these medications, if in his judgment they are indicated. But medical experts add some warnings here. No patient should ever take them unsupervised, nor should he have the druggist renew them without the doctor's permission.

If you suffer from an ulcer or from tuberculosis or from any other chronic disease, make sure the doctor knows about these conditions if he contemplates giving you any cortisone-like drug or ACTH internally. If the physician plans to give them to you over a prolonged period—more than ten days, let us say—make sure that he follows your blood pressure and takes a chest X ray. If you develop any ankle swelling, indigestion, or weight loss while using these drugs, your doctor should be informed immediately.

## Why Don't You Speak for Yourself, Dale Alexander?

Now—let's get on to *my* recommendations.

My experience makes me believe most wholeheartedly in diet as the primary treatment for seborrhea of the scalp and for thinning hair and baldness. As I kept close track of my own problem, I found that the hair and scalp were harmfully affected by hydrogenated fats like butter and the older margarines and by fat that had been subjected to high heat as in frying—especially deep-fat frying, as in the preparation of potato chips and French fried potatoes. I am against salted foods for the same reason. I particularly object to foods such as salted roasted peanuts, roasted corn chips, tacos, and the like. I avoid these like the plague, being utterly convinced that they are injurious to the hair. I don't know the *physiology* of the harmfulness of salted foods—but of the *result* I have no doubt.

As to shampooing, I believe in soapless shampoos used daily, if that is necessary to keep the scalp clean. Especially avoid a harsh tincture or green soap, which contains alcohol that may stimulate the sebaceous glands to give forth even more sebum. Nor do I believe in castile shampoos, which are based on coconut oil, the most heavily saturated of all the vegetable oils. In my opinion, the soapless shampoos do a better job of cleaning than any other type of shampoo available; I think this is easily demonstrable. Just wash your hair one day with a soapless shampoo and another day with a castile shampoo. With the former, your hair will feel finer and silkier. If you scratch your scalp with your fingernail after each shampoo, you will find more loose scales remaining on your scalp after the castile shampoo than you will after the soapless shampoo.

I believe in thorough brushing with a natural bristle brush. Nylon bristles may split the hairs. Avoid over-brushing of areas where the hair is very fine—that is, areas where new hairs are growing in or old, unhealthy ones are ready to break off or fall out. I do not believe in hair tonics, "restorers," dandruff removers, dyes, curling solutions, straightening pomades, or anything else that provides an artificial solution.

I believe that sufficient vitamins can be obtained from a well-chosen diet. In extreme cases, supplementation with various B vitamins may be helpful. I do not believe in rubbing anything into the hair or scalp in the form of an ointment or cream, except what may be prescribed by a skin doctor. The dermatologist will usually prescribe sulfur, resorcin, or coal-tar in one form or another—old remedies that, as any dermatologist will admit, leave much to be desired. Certainly they are sometimes effective, but often only temporarily.

To summarize, I believe in diet, cleanliness, and commonsense care.

# 8

# MY THIRTY-YEAR SEARCH—AND THE BOOK THAT STARTED ME ON THE RIGHT TRACK

I have told you of my old anguish, as a teenager, over the loss of my hair and the teasing I was forced to take. I didn't realize at the time that this cloud would have a silver lining—that is, the opportunity to impart to others knowledge that has helped me.

I ran the gamut of drugstore remedies, folk remedies, friends' advice—but all to no avail. I tried rubbing my scalp with lanolin (also called hydrous wool fat) because it was an animal fat and, theoretically, should mix better with human tissue than a mineral grease like vaseline. It didn't help; my brother claimed I smelled more like a sheep than a human.

While reading about lanolin, I stumbled across the fact that the weight of wool a sheep grows is controlled by the amount and quality of the food it consumes. A poor diet reduces the breaking strength and the length and diameter of wool fibers. M. L. Ryder, of the Wool Industries Research Association, located in Leeds, England, has shown that reinforcement of the diet with both protein and carbohydrate corrects these defects and increases wool production. Apparently the carbohydrate is needed to provide energy to utilize the protein and to allow the protein to be used for wool formation rather than itself being used for energy, as happens when the diet is carbohydrate-poor.

Bullough and Laurence, of the University of London, convincingly demonstrated that carbohydrate is essential to growth in the hair follicle. Oxygen is also necessary. But this discussion of the growing follicle's need for carbohydrate left me with a dilemma. If the growing follicle needs carbohydrate, why did my hair cease to grow when I was on a carbohydrate-rich diet? I was forced to conclude that the process of *refining* sugar removes some unknown substance or substances which are helpful to hair growth.

I tried dowsing my hair with hot olive oil; I tried vinegar. My brother told me to mix the two, and add salt and pepper, bottle and sell the mixture, and use the money received to buy myself a wig. It was a crude joke, but it emphasized to me that I had made no progress whatsoever under this regimen. When I added an egg shampoo to my program, my brother really howled. Unknowingly, he gave me good advice. "Eat them, don't waste good eggs on your thick skull," was his fraternal comment.

Years later, when I had delved into this subject, I remembered his remark and wished I had taken it seriously. I was to learn that the keratin of the cortex of the hair, as has been shown by Wilkerson and confirmed by Block, contains a very high sulfur content; eggs are a prime source of sulfur in the human diet. I believe that eggs should be eaten *raw* because cooking will kill the germinal center of a fertilized egg; and I believe that wherever possible, *fertilized eggs* should be used. The fertilized egg is an important "germinating" food in my diet.

## The Inside-Out Approach

I finally concluded .that my head was not like my automobile—it didn't benefit from oiling and greasing from the *outside*. The proper oils for the hair had to be produced from the *inside*, from the substances brought to the sebaceous glands of the scalp by the bloodstream. And *now*, all I had to do was find out which substances nourished the hair follicles, which stimulated them to grow, and which provided sustenance for the sebaceous glands. That was all! It took me only a few years to formulate the questions—but it took almost three decades to find the answers.

In the intervening time, I had the depressing experience of being mistaken for my girl friend's father. "Forty," her chum said, "forty if he's a day." And I was twenty-two! I took to wearing a baseball cap or a beret; I even contemplated becoming a sikh by adoption so that I could cover my lack of hair with a turban.

One fine day it occurred to me that my twin brother, Morrie, had a fine head of glossy black hair. I begged him to tell me the secret; he insisted there was none. The more I pestered him for an answer, the more obdurate he became. I decided to study him secretly. The only difference I could notice between his way of life and mine—now, don't laugh—was that he ate the onions on his hamburgers raw and I liked mine fried! At first I ignored this "silly" finding. Then I realized that he not only ate raw hamburger onions; he ate all kinds of raw onions—Bermuda, Spanish, spring—you name them and Morrie devoured them.

I studied the onion. I found that 100 grams of raw onion has almost three times the amount of protein, twice the amount of carbohydrate, and twice as much vitamins A, B, and C as 100 grams of cooked onion. I found that green spring onions were an excellent source of vitamin C. I found that potassium, the mineral that is so important in intracellular metabolism, is found in large quantities in the raw onion. "Aha," I said to myself, "I have found the answer!" I began to eat even more raw onions than Morrie. I carried scallions in waxed paper in my pocket. What did it matter that the Alexander boys were losing all their friends? I felt that, if only I could regain my lost locks, I could again win friends and influence people. And for a time I felt as though I were making "headway." My hair loss seemed to slow down. But I soon realized that onions were not the whole story, for the thinning continued, though at a slightly lessened rate.

I continued to study Morrie, and anyone else in a cafeteria or a restaurant who possessed a good head of hair. Strangers fidgeted uneasily under the gaze of that young man who eyed their food trays, then began to scribble furiously in a pocket notebook. I studied the dietary habits of persons with bald heads. I also studied my own eating habits—wondering, for instance, why my rate of hair loss increased in the summer months and decreased in the winter. I watched chefs at work and read cookbooks, eventually becoming something of an expert on the subject of food preparation. When I started, I didn't know a *coupe St. Jacques* from a *coquille St. Jacques.* I picked up information from whatever source I could. One of the most useful was Dione Lucas' *Gourmet Cooking School Cookbook.*

From such books I learned not only how to cook but also how to arrange attractively the simple foods I finally selected as the ideal diet for my hair's health. Using Dione Lucas' recipe for the *salade simple* as a basis, I evolved the Alexander Salad, a major item in my program to promote the NuGrow Cycle. The recipe for the salad appears in Chapter Ten.

### Turning Point

Then I was lucky enough to happen upon a book that confirmed all my slowly gathered knowledge. If only I had known of it when I first became interested in dietary control of hair growth, I might have saved myself years of study.

Several years ago, as was my wont, I was browsing through some old medical texts in a New England library. The title of one of them brought me up short:

HAIR
*Its Nature, Growth and Most Common Affections*
*with*
*Hygienic Rules for its Preservation*
*by*
*Dr. Richard Muller*

Since this book had been written as long ago as 1913, I was going to pass it by, but some sixth sense made me open it. As I thumbed through it, I became more and more fascinated. Here was a researcher, eminent in his time, who had not only studied the skin and hair under the distinguished Sabouraud in Paris but had also continued his learning at the leading institutions of London, Vienna, and Berlin.

His conclusions, which I quote, were almost identical with mine. In a chapter called "On Food in General and Especially for the Growth of Hair," he states: "The growth of hair depends entirely on the blood supply. Anemic, sclerotic, exhausted, ill-nourished people will grow no hair while their condition is below normal. . . . To make blood, food is needed, food in proper amounts and proper quality." He cited Dr. Lucien Jacques, an eminent French dermatologist who, in 1910, noticed that a number of patients at the Saint-Antoine Hospital had suffered serious hair loss. Yet he could find no local scalp disease nor any systemic disease to account for the hair loss. Jacques asked his assistant, Dr. Henri Buillard, to study these patients carefully for two years—not only what they did to their hair and scalps, but *all* their habits.

The result of this detailed investigation of seventy-one patients made a volume of some 400 pages and included heretofore unreported findings. Each of these patients suffered from some disorder of the alimentary tract. The majority of them ate too fast and did not chew their food sufficiently, with the result that it was not properly mixed with the saliva. They also drank excessive quantities of alcohol, coffee, and tea. Instead of eating and chewing carefully, they bolted their food. The good doctors then induced them to change their eating habits. A dramatic change was seen. "New hair grew!" That phrase leaped out at me. *New hair grew!*

*Now* I read avidly everything Muller had to say. He compared the human body to an engine and the stomach to its boiler. He felt that it was important to stoke the boiler with foods that would nourish the various organs of the body. Food that did not nourish the body he likened to ashes and clinkers. To make blood that was good for nourishing the hair, Muller recommended milk, cheese, eggs, and fish. He believed that the milk should be heated to 100 degrees Fahrenheit and sipped slowly on an empty stomach. Apparently, milk taken that way would not chill and constrict the blood vessels of the stomach and small intestine and so not interfere with the circulation to the digestive glands. We know now, of course, that iced drinks may so interfere with the circulation that they will produce a noticeable change in the electrocardiogram; a large meal may do the same thing. But Muller's book was written eleven years before William Einthoven received the Nobel Prize for inventing the electrocardiograph! Muller's conclusion was based on sheer clinical acumen.

## The Egg's the Thing

When he discussed eggs, he stressed that they must be fresh and raw. I agree, but for different reasons. Dr. Muller believed that fresh raw eggs are digested more than twice as fast as the cooked variety. Doctors today have learned that this is not wholly true. We realize by now that cooking is a sort of first step in the digestive process of proteins; cooking begins, and the digestive enzymes complete, the "reprocessing" of protein to proteoses, polypeptides, and finally to the amino acids that the body uses for building new tissues. In that regard, cooking eggs might be considered beneficial. However, it is obvious that our gastrointestinal systems can digest the *white* of the egg without any trouble, cooked or uncooked. With the *yolk* of the egg—a fat— the story is not so clear. Polymerization of fats, produced by the heat of cooking, may result in a marked reduction in their digestibility. Heated fats show increased viscosity and changes in their intimate chemical structure.

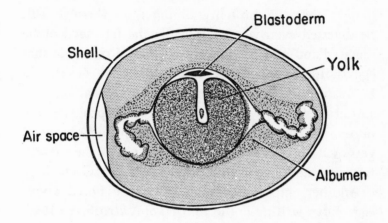

Shell · Blastoderm · Yolk · Air space · Albumen

## THE FERTILE EGG, SOURCE OF HAIR NOURISHMENT

Fresh raw fertile eggs are a prime source of germinative components, contributing to the growth factors so necessary to initiate the Nu-Grow Cycle described in Chapter Eight.

*A.* The shell—an excellent source of calcium.

*B.* The yolk—a source of fat.

*C.* The white, which contains albumen, a protein.

*D.* The blastoderm or embryo.

Crampton and others, writing in the *Journal of Nutrition* in 1951, reported that efficiency of diets containing fats polymerized by heat was decreased below that of similar diets containing unheated fats. Since I believe that the protein (albumen) of the egg will be digested even when raw while the fat may not be digested and may pass out in the stool, I conclude that eggs should be eaten *raw*. I also believe that eggs should be *fresh and fertile*. Fresh, raw, fertile eggs, along with sprouting foods (with the exception of sprouting potatoes, which are dangerous), are a prime source of germinative components, contributing to the growth factors so necessary to initiate the NuGrow Cycle.

Another important point should be noted about eggs. Burr, writing in the *Journal of Nutrition* in 1944, was the first to point out that fats are digested to a lesser extent on a low-protein regimen than on a high-protein diet. Several other investigators have confirmed these findings. An egg consists of three chief constituents: albumen (protein), yolk (fat), and shell (calcium). Since investigators have shown that calcium *decreases* the digestibility of fats, I have not suggested throwing the entire egg, shell and all, in a blender as is done in some diets. But I do maintain that a raw, fresh, fertile egg contains many of the chief components of a hair-nourishing diet, including large amounts of vitamins A and D.

It is of great interest that Deuel, in Volume II of *The Lipids,* published in 1955, shows that fats have a slightly higher digestibility in the female than in the male. Could this be connected with the fact that the female keeps her hair longer than does the male? It seems to make sense.

To return to Dr. Muller, he anticipated modern investigators by stating that sugar was an excellent food. Bullough, as recently as the early 1950s, demonstrated that sugar is necessary for the growth of hair. But Bullough's work was done on the *rat*, while I observed human beings. And in human beings I must conclude that honey, molasses, and other unrefined sugars do not interfere with hair growth, while refined white sugar, as found in ice cream, candy, and pop, and on the average dining table, does so interfere.

Muller's diet for promoting the growth of hair was interesting. He advised the consumption of raw eggs, carrots, oatmeal, toasted bread, raw milk, gelatin, and a soup made of two parts of meat and one part of bones. How he arrived at this diet is intriguing. Apparently, he was influenced by the homeopathic view prevalent at the time. Simply stated, it is *similia similibus curantur*—that is, diseases are cured (or should be treated) by those drugs which produce symptoms similar to them in the healthy. If a patient suffered from a running nose, for example, one was supposed to give him minute doses of a drug that made the nose run.

Muller included in his diet those foods that contained chemicals similar to those contained in the hair. This reasoning was accepted in his day, but it doesn't go far enough. Muller's knowledge of the anatomy of the hair follicle did not include the refinements imparted to us by the electron microscope. He had no notion of the importance of vitamins, of the physiology of the resting and active phases of hair growth, of the chemistry of keratinization, of the effects of the different hormones. After all, hormones weren't even discovered until about 1921.

Muller knew that carrots had traditionally been given to horses to help them produce a fine coat and mane. His diet and his reasoning intrigued me. I tried raw carrots with minor success. (I had noticed that brother Morrie nibbled on raw carrots between meals.) With a great effort of will, I added raw eggs to my diet and again noted an improvement.

## What about the Palate?

But how to improve the taste and consistency of raw eggs? About this time, I became interested in so-called health foods. These are foods eaten regularly in other parts of the world but neglected in our own Western culture. The subtle, nutlike flavor of wheat germ intrigued me even before I realized that it possessed valuable germinating properties. I mixed it with the raw eggs in a blender and found the resulting concoction more palatable than raw eggs alone. And then I was introduced to wheat germ oil, which, I felt, contained all the valuable properties of the wheat germ and, in addition, the hair-promoting and nourishing attributes of a good vegetable oil. I tried these and other foods alone, in combinations, and prepared in various ways. I began to weed out foods that didn't help me or actually seemed to harm. I added any food that seemed to help. I finally formulated a dietary program of hair growth, as well as the concept of the NuGrow Cycle. I am happy to acknowledge my debt to Dr. Richard Muller, that pioneer in the field of the dietary treatment of falling hair.

# 9

# THE HAIR COCKTAIL: THE WAY TO A MAN'S HEAD IS THROUGH HIS STOMACH

I know what you've been thinking: okay, you've convinced me that diet is the key to a healthy head of hair. Okay, you've taught me all I need to know about the medical background of the subject. Now when do we get to the real substance of the course, Professor Alexander?

The answer is: here and now. But remember, if we hadn't gone through the essential preliminaries, none of this would hold the meaning for you that it can and will.

Our first specific step toward the objective you are eager to achieve is the Alexander Hair Cocktail. Most cocktails will addle your pate, but this one grew hair on mine! Most cocktails make you *feel* like a new man, but this will help you *be* one. So bottoms up to a new top!

Let me give you some rules for making and taking the Alexander blockbuster; then I'll give you a short, scientific explanation of why I advise such attention to details.

## HOW TO MAKE AND TAKE THE ALEXANDER HAIR COCKTAIL

You will need an electric blender. This need not be an expensive one. The cheaper ones made of plexiglass, readily available in most appliance, health food, and department stores, will do just as well.

1. Take three-quarters of a glass of whole milk. This should preferably be raw certified milk. However, if that is not available, regular homogenized cow's milk will do. Pour the milk into the blender.

2. Add one raw egg to the milk in the blender. This should preferably be a fertile egg. But if fertile eggs cannot be secured, use regularly available fresh eggs.

3. Add one tablespoonful of raw wheat germ oil.

4. Add two tablespoonsful of raw wheat germ. Do not use the toasted variety.

5. Add one tablespoonful each of the three seed meals: Sunflower, pumpkin, and sesame meals. Also add one tablespoonful of Chia seeds. To this, add one ripe banana or one piece of your favorite fresh fruit. The seed meals, as well as the Chia seeds, are generally available in health food stores. These are the germanating substances and are critically important.

6. Blend at low speed from two to three minutes.

7. Drink this blended mixture promptly.

8. This drink should serve as your complete breakfast.

9. Do not eat or drink anything else for two hours after taking this mixture.

10. The wheat germ oil, milk, and eggs used in this drink should be kept under refrigeration at all times. The raw wheat germ should be kept in a sealed container, preferably under refrigeration.

Do not supplement the wheat germ oil you take in this drink with wheat germ oil capsules during the day.

Once you notice changes in your hair, you may cut down on the daily intake of the hair cocktail and take it only twice a week. Of course, since it is a healthful drink, you may prefer to continue taking it daily indefinitely.

## The Wheat Germ Oil and Milk Mixture—A Modified Version of the Hair Cocktail

Now there are some people who may prefer to take another blend, which is a modified but still potent version of the hair cocktail. This is a mixture of wheat germ oil and milk.

For people who have the four problems listed below, this mixture is a suitable alternative:

1. They are allergic to eggs, or do not like to eat them raw.

2. They are trying to cut down on their calories.

3. They have hair that is very dry, and need a mixture that will enhance its luster.

4. They have been told to limit their egg intake by their physicians.

It is also a good idea for those who take the hair cocktail as a complete breakfast to supplement it with this second mixture at night half an hour before retiring.

### How to Mix and Take the Oil and Milk Cocktail

You will need some whole milk, some wheat germ oil, a tablespoon, and a small screw-top jar, if you have no blender.

1. Put six tablespoonsful of whole milk into the jar or blender.

2. Add one tablespoonful of virgin, cold-pressed wheat germ oil to the milk. Cover and shake or blend for ten to fifteen seconds. You will notice hundreds of tiny oil bubbles. (For even better results, put the ingredients into a blender and homogenize for ten to fifteen seconds.)

3. Drink the mixture immediately.

4. The optimal method of taking the mixture is to drink it about thirty minutes before breakfast. If the mixture is taken at night, drink it at least four

hours after the evening meal. For best results, the stomach should be empty.

5. Keep your bottle of wheat germ oil refrigerated at all times to prevent it from becoming rancid.

6. It is advisable to use a small jar when mixing the ingredients. If you use a large jar, more oil will be left clinging to the inside surfaces of the jar, and your hair will receive less. If you use a blender, which I recommend, use six ounces of milk rather than six tablespoonsful; but the amount of wheat germ oil you mix with it remains the same.

7. *Do not mix the wheat germ oil with lemon or grapefruit juice.* You may use fresh, strained orange juice. Whole sweet milk is the best liquid available for mixing. Those who do not care for sweet milk may substitute soybean milk.

8. Do not use nonfat milk.

9. Do not use wheat germ oil capsules in place of bottled oil.

10. After a certain period of time, you should start to taper down on the use of the wheat germ oil mixture. When? Cut down when you see that the dryness of your hair and scalp has been corrected, when your hairfall has been alleviated, when you see that your hair has become glossy. But do not stop the intake of wheat germ oil suddenly. Keep taking the mixture every other morning, instead of daily. Continue this plan for approximately

three months. Then use the oil at least twice each month.

11. Take the wheat germ oil alone without the milk if you wish. It has other advantages. It is a good supply of energy for the body. But for optimal hair results, consume the wheat germ oil mixed with whole sweet milk.

The above rules on how to take the wheat germ oil mixture apply to the millions of people who have hair-fall problems. They also apply to anyone and everyone who wants to avoid *future* hairfall problems. This mixture is designed to reverse and stop abnormal hairfall. It is not designed to regrow hair, however. The mixture is particularly beneficial for people with thinning hair. They have hair to work with.

People who already have more than 25 percent hair loss need a much more extensive hair rehabilitation program. They also need the hair cocktail and skilled professional hair attention and guidance. If you are more than 75 percent bald, it is now a question whether you have fuzz to work with or if your scalp is already too tight. If the scalp is skintight, it is almost hopeless to attempt to regrow hair. My program works best for partially balding people rather than for those already bald.. But even the latter would be wise to follow the complete program. It is designed to help the entire body as well as the hair. Falling hair is not just a scalp problem; it is a constitutional problem.

The only exceptions to the eleven rules on mixing

wheat germ oil are for people having other illnesses along with their abnormal hairfall. Anyone suffering from gallbladder trouble, high blood pressure, heart trouble, hardening of the arteries, or stroke should consult a physician before trying this mixture. Also those with special allergies to wheat products should see a physician before trying this program. Fortunately, they are few.

## Special Wheat Germ Oil Rules for Special Situations

Those who work late shifts or unusual hours can consume the wheat germ oil mixture at times convenient to their working schedule and sleeping hours. It may be taken at whatever hour you arise, just so it is taken about half an hour before the first meal and at least half an hour after any water intake. Or it can be imbibed just before going to sleep, at least four hours after any intake. Or if necessary, it can be taken just before leaving for work, providing it has been four hours since eating and at least half an hour before any new food is to be eaten.

Anyone, with the exceptions noted above, may take the wheat germ oil mixture as an aid to the reproductive qualities of his or her hair. Once a week is enough, after a two- to three-month period of daily consumption, if the hair and scalp are dry. The once-a-week routine is a maintenance program.

The majority of people will find the mixture very easy to take.

## Fat Absorption

Now let's consider the reasons for these rules. We must start with a modicum of physiology, just a few lines on the absorption of fats and the factors that affect this absorption.

First of all, no digestion of fats takes place in the mouth. There is a certain amount of separation of fats from other foods that takes place in the stomach, a necessary prerequisite to their digestion and absorption in the small intestine.

This separation is due to the beginnings of the breakdown of proteins through the action of pepsin, an enzyme formed by the walls of the stomach, plus the breakdown of starches due to the enzyme ptyalin, which comes from the saliva and mixes with the food in the stomach. There may be a small amount of fat digestion in the stomach, possibly due to a little lipase, a fat-digesting enzyme from the pancreas, leaking back through the small intestine into the stomach; the evidence is unclear and the amount is unimportant. The food remains in the stomach for a time that is roughly proportionate to the amount of fat in the intake. When the amount of fat taken in is large, the food stays in the stomach longer. The average stay in the stomach is between two and four hours. It then enters the small intestine.

The pancreatic lipase enzyme called steapsin now does most of the digesting of fats. It is secreted in the pancreatic juice. It is aided by the bile, which not only

| ENZYME | WHAT IT BREAKS DOWN |
|--------|---------------------|
| Pepsin | Protein |
| Ptyalin | Starches |
| Lipase | Fats |
| Steapsin (aided by bile) | Major digester of fats (frees fatty acids) |

## ENZYMES AND THEIR FUNCTIONS

Enzymes are proteins, produced by cells, which have the power to initiate or accelerate specific chemical reactions in the metabolism of plants and animals. The various enzymes, as shown in the chart, break down and separate starches, proteins, and fats for easier absorption into the bloodstream. Since the blood directly contributes to the health of the hair root, the importance of the function of these enzymes cannot be overstated.

emulsifies the fat, making smaller fat globules with decreased surface tension that are more easily attacked by the steapsin, but probably also helps produce the right amount of alkalinity for the action of the steapsin. The combined action of bile and steapsin results in breakdown of the fat to free fatty acids. And then, as the fatty acids are absorbed through the intestinal wall, they are recombined, finally forming tryglycerides, also known as neutral fats. These neutral fats go via the lymphatic vessels of the intestinal wall, known as lacteals, to the general lymphatic system and thence into the blood stream, and so to the capillary network of the hair follicles.

It is now believed that little or no absorption of fats occurs in the large intestine. In fact, there is actually some secretion of fats into the large intestine, these fats then being lost in fecal material.

In general, animal and vegetable fats are well absorbed and well digested by the human being. The higher the melting point of fats, the less efficiently they are utilized. Wheat germ oil has an extremely low melting point and is very well absorbed and digested. Another type of lipid, cholesterol, is present in large quantities in the yolks of eggs. This has been shown to be better absorbed in the human being in the presence of another fat than it is alone. Therefore, I suggest the use of wheat germ oil together with eggs and the butterfat of milk as a well-absorbed, well-utilized lipid combination.

Incidentally, scientists express this idea in what they term the "coefficient of digestibility." The formula is to take the fat ingested minus the fat excreted (corrected for metabolized fat), divide this by the amount of fat ingested and multiply the result by 100. Butter has a coefficient of 97, as opposed to mutton fat with a coefficient of 88 or deer fat with a coefficient of only 81.7. This means that butterfat is well digested.

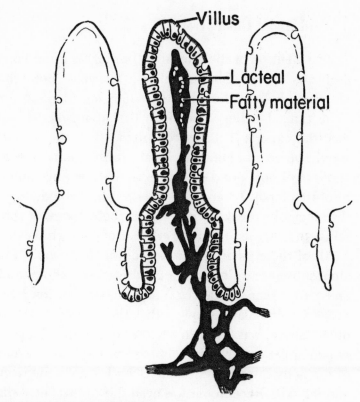

**Villus**

**Lacteal**

**Fatty material**

## CROSS-SECTION OF VILLI

Villi are small finger-like projections of the mucosa (mucous membrane) into the small intestine. These projections contain the lymphatic vessels known as lacteals. The lacteals carry neutral fats, already broken down by the activity of the enzymes, to the general lymphatic system, which in turn carries the fats through the bloodstream and on to the papillae, or capillary network, at the hair root. Thus it is the villi that may be called the transfer point of the neutral fats from the digestive system into the bloodstream. Their contribution to healthy hair is, therefore, of great importance.

## A Word About Cholesterol

The mention of cholesterol will probably cause some eyebrows to rise. Cholesterol and fats have been the whipping boys of the popular writers on nutrition for some time. I believe, based on the advice of the top medical experts I have consulted, that the record should be set straight. First of all, in the human body, cholesterol does not derive directly from eating cholesterol-rich foods. It can be synthesized in the body from the metabolic breakdown of fats, carbohydrates, or proteins—in fact, even from the ethyl alcohol of whiskey.

All of these foods are broken down to a two-carbon atom substance called acetate; and from this cholesterol and many other substances are synthesized. As long ago as 1952, Alfin-Slater showed that the rate of synthesis of cholesterol was uniform whether or not the diet contained no fat or as much as 30 percent fat. Many tissues of the body can synthesize cholesterol, chiefly the liver and the skin. Recently, it was even shown that the walls of the body's largest artery, the aorta, could synthesize cholesterol.

Despite variations in the amount of cholesterol in the diet, the bodily tissues maintain themselves at a uniform cholesterol level in a healthy body. Vigorous attempts to lower the cholesterol level of the blood by rigorously restricting cholesterol and fat intake not only fail in a large percentage of cases but actually entail other dangers. For example, in the absence of fat in the diet, abnormally large amounts of cholesterol accumulate in the liver of experimental rats, in spite of a lowering of the blood cholesterol to unusually low levels.

On the other hand, fats have great protective value. If calories are needed for warmth, for growth, or for any other purpose, fat will supply by far the greatest number of calories. Fats are usually thought of as containing nine calories to every four for protein or carbohydrate. However, this does not take into consideration that our food, as we eat it, usually presents us with proteins and carbohydrates diluted with a measurable quantity of water, while fat is ordinarily water-free. And calories *are* necessary—for the many chemical processes occurring in all of us at all times. Fats make the diet more palatable. Fats help the body use the B-vitamin, thiamine. Fats carry the fat-soluble vitamins A, D, and K.

Fats also help the body save valuable protein. Experiments show that human beings fed on *low* fat diets lost nitrogen, the end results of protein breakdown, in their urine instead of using it for tissue building, as they did when fed a *high* fat diet. Rats grow best when their diets contain 30 percent fat. Fat shows what is termed an "associative dynamic action." That is, when plentiful amounts of fat are present in the diet, the heat loss induced by protein and carbohydrate metabolism almost disappears, suggesting that these heat calories are being used instead of wasted. (Incidentally, this might indicate that one way to stay cooler in the summer is to eat plenty of fat with each meal.) Finally, work capacity is lessened by a fat-free diet.

## What Kinds of Fats to Eat

There are three so-called essential fatty acids, that is, fatty acids that are necessary for nutrition but that cannot be manufactured by the body on its own and must therefore be included in the diet. The first two, linoleic acid and linolenic acid, are obtained from vegetable oils. The third, arachidonic acid, is found exclusively in animal fats. Infants on a low-fat diet may develop eczema, which is easily cured by feeding them fat. Although attempts have been made to implicate high fat intake as the cause of hardening of the arteries, the evidence at this writing is far from convincing. Even the so-called prudent diet, conceived by the late Dr. Norman Jolliffe and his disciples, allows four eggs per week and plentiful fats from poultry and fish.

The evidence seems to be accumulating that the American diet is too high in calories, and possibly too high in saturated fats—that is, fats obtained from mutton, lamb, veal, pork, and beef—and too low in the less saturated fats—those from poultry and fish and shellfish. I believe that the best way to lower your caloric intake is to eliminate cake, ice cream, soda pop, and candy, all made with refined white sugar and containing little or no essential ingredients.

If you have a family history of, or yourself suffer

| UNSATURATED FATS | SATURATED FATS |
|---|---|
| Shell Fish | Beef, Pork |
| Fish | Veal |
| Poultry | Lamb |

The popular diet with modern physicians is the high unsaturated fat, low saturated fat, low cholesterol diet. This can be achieved by stressing the foods listed above under "Unsaturated Fats" and de-emphasizing the "Saturated Fats."

from high blood pressure, heart or blood-vessel trouble, or stroke, you would do well to get your physician's opinion before embarking on my program's commitment to one egg daily. Even so, however, I predict that your physician will sanction my diet. If, after a breakfast of an Alexander Hair Cocktail, your other two meals stress poultry and fish and shellfish and eliminate as far as possible sheep, cattle, and pig fats, you will be eating a diet that contains predominantly polyunsaturated fats and yet is, in my opinion, still nourishing to the hair follicles.

Don't forget that cholesterol is the basic substance from which almost all our hormones are made. Choles-

terol in the skin is the source of vitamin $D_3$, after irradiation of the skin by sunlight or an ultraviolet lamp.
In the liver, cholesterol is converted into the bile acids,
essential ingredients of the bile. So not only is it impossible for one to rid his body entirely of cholesterol,
it would be disastrous if it could be accomplished. One
of the hair dressings referred to as "greasy kid stuff"
used to boast on its label that it contained cholesterol.
When cholesterol became unstylish, that word disap-
peared from its label.

### Drawing a Few Conclusions

One last thought about fats. It is known that the
character of the fat in a body can be changed by diet.
For example, in the 1920s in this country, farmers and
consumers suffered from the "soft-pork" problem. The
fat in the carcasses of hogs that had received a diet containing large proportions of soybeans or peanuts was so
soft that the slabs of bacon were shapeless and, therefore, worthless. It was found that the lard in these slabs
of bacon contained large quantities of linoleic acid
from the beans or peanuts in the diet. When other
types of fats replaced some of the fat containing linoleic
acid, the bacon again became firm and easier to handle.
The thing that hardened the lard most efficiently was
found to be a high carbohydrate diet. Now comes my
own contention—unproven so far except by my experiments on myself. I have found that a diet high in polyunsaturated fats in proportion to saturated fats and low

in carbohydrates produces a sebum that is more liquid and therefore more easily washed from the scalp. Therefore, I used this type of diet and found it most helpful in eradicating my bald spots and adding gloss to my formerly dull mop.

Why do I suggest using a blender to mix my recommended recipes? In a blender, the oil and egg yolk take on the form of millions of tiny droplets too fine to be seen with the naked eye. These droplets present much more surface for the digestive enzymes to work on than does the unblended food.

Why do I insist on refrigeration? Steenbock, in 1936, showed that rancid fat is more slowly absorbed than fresh fat; so we want to keep our fat fresh and wholesome.

Why do I prefer raw milk to pasteurized milk? As I have mentioned earlier in the book, fats subject to heat are more slowly digested than fats not subject to heat. During the process of pasteurization, the fats in milk are subjected to either 143 degrees Fahrenheit for thirty minutes or 160 degrees Fahrenheit for fifteen seconds. Raw milk is not subjected to these high temperatures. (Remember, I am recommending *certified* raw milk for safety.)

A similar objection holds for the wheat germ, which contains ten grams of oil for every 100 grams of wheat germ. Why make this less digestible by heating it?

Why drink it immediately? Two reasons: (1) drink it before the oil globules can coalesce, making them less digestible; (2) drink it before the fats can become rancid.

Why eat nothing with it? So that there will be less separating for the stomach to do, and so that the digestive process in the intestine will be easier. Also, the presence of fat in the stomach slows its emptying time; if other foods are present with these fats, the former will not get out of the stomach as fast and may make you feel uncomfortably heavy.

Now you know how to make the hair cocktail, how to protect the integrity of its ingredients, why I believe in it, and its exact preparation. All that's left for you to do is—try it!

# 10

# SEVEN DAYS OF
# HAIR-NOURISHING MENUS
# FOR THREE KINDS OF
# HAIR PROBLEMS

Now we come to the "meat of the matter"—
*and* the vegetables, *and* the fruits—to help readers with
their hair problems. I have provided three sets of
menus for persons with three different degrees of hair
difficulty: those who suffer from thinning hair, those
with relatively little scalp hair, and those with annoy-
ing dandruff. I offer suggestions for three meals daily
for a week in each category, and rely upon the reader
to recombine and substitute similarly nourishing foods
for the subsequent weeks. You will find it becomes an
enjoyable game, choosing for oneself foods that not
only benefit the depressed hair follicle but look and
taste fresh and fine. And in the modern home equipped
with an electric blender but not servants, they are easy
and quick to prepare.

121

1. For persons with thinning hair, I have emphasized the hair cocktail and the Alexander Salad. These bring to the diet a rich supply of vitamins, proteins, and minerals, thus providing for each hair follicle its optimal chemical environment.

2. For those whose hair is almost gone, I suggest more of the germinating foods, such as the milk shake fortified with germinating seeds, the liberal use of vegetable and grain sprouts and chia seed pudding. This type of dietary enrichment will, I am sure, increase the reproductive potential of the cells of the hair follicles and offer the needed nutrients for new hair growth.

3. Lastly comes dandruff. It is my firm opinion that this distressing condition can be immeasurably aided by large amounts of naturally occurring vitaman B. My menus, therefore, feature the vitamin B milk shake, my own concoction, which consists of brewer's yeast, desiccated liver, and raw wheat germ. The desiccated liver, by the way, is merely dried liver that has been granulated and can be blended easily with other ingredients. You will notice that the use of white sugar has been eliminated completely; I consider this essential to a successful diet.

Many of the foods and supplements listed in this chapter must be bought in health food stores, since they are not carried by the corner grocery or the local supermarket. I consider this a sad commentary on the state of the American diet. Such worthwhile nutriment should occupy the places on the shelves of groceries now occupied by white bread, refined flour, white sugar, and white rice. Wives and mothers of the world, unite! You have nothing to lose but your chins! Demand chia! Demand wheat germ! Demand brown sugar! Demand equal representation!

Please be sure to follow these rules in preparing your own menus:

1. Take the hair cocktail as your breakfast each morning. The longer you continue with the hair cocktail as your first meal, the better for your hair.

2. If you do not take the hair cocktail as your breakfast, then you definitely should take the optional wheat germ oil and milk mixture. This will make certain that you are getting some of the nutrients you have missed at breakfast.

2. If you eat sweets or desserts, stick to those made with natural products—for example, pies made with brown sugar, fresh fruit, and whole wheat crusts. You may also eat salads of fresh fruit and yogurt and milk shakes made of yogurt and fruit juice.

4. If you must have something to nibble on between meals, take sunflower seeds, which are quite palatable, pumpkin seeds, raisins, macadamia nuts, or

any unroasted, unsalted nuts such as cashews and filberts, or celery or carrot sticks.

5. It is extremely important to stress salads composed largely of greens. In any hair rebuilding program, the tossed green salad is *second in importance only to the hair cocktail.* On many evenings it can even serve as the entire meal along with a glass of milk. The proper preparation of greens plays such a major role in my NuGrow Cycle that I've devised my own personal recipe.

## The Alexander Salad

I feel certain you'll love the Alexander Salad. Everyone who's ever tasted it has raved about it. Recently, during a talent show at Patsy D'Amore's famous Villa Capri restaurant in Hollywood, I made the salad for forty people. It was a smash hit. Everybody clamored for second helpings. The maître d' was so excited by the salad's unique flavor that he took a portion home to share it with his wife. It was the talk of the restaurant for weeks afterward.

Another good thing about this delicious and nutritious salad is that it goes a long way. If you prepare the salad as described below, it will easily serve a family of four. Moreover, if there is any left over, it will keep for days in the refrigerator. The lemon juice helps to keep it fresh.

## How to Make the Alexander Salad

INGREDIENTS

green parsley

green watercress

green romaine lettuce

green onions including
  shoots

red sweet onions

greenish alfalfa sprouts

beige Jerusalem
  artichokes

baby carrots

red cabbage

green cucumbers

green zucchini

green celery

green or red pepper

golden raw sweet corn

red tomatoes

SEASONINGS

oregano

lemon concentrate
  powder

orange concentrate
  powder

lemon juice

almond meal

choice of oil made from
  sunflower seeds,
  safflower seeds, or
  soybeans

enzyme seasoning

organic mineral powder

(The last two items are generally available only in health food shops but can be specially ordered in other food stores.)

Wash and clean all vegetables. Do not remove outside skin layers of any vegetables except the red onion and sweet corn. Remember that all vegetables used must be served in their raw state.

You will need an oversized wooden salad bowl and large wooden spoon and fork. Since this is a salad of layer upon layer of greens designed to distribute oils effectively and to mask the odors of the onions, please follow mixing and tossing directions very carefully.

Take one-third of a bunch of green parsley. Cut up into quarter-inch-long segments. Place pieces in bowl. Do same with one-third of a bunch of green watercress. Toss parsley and watercress in bowl.

Take ten to twelve leaves of green romaine lettuce. Cut up in half-inch segments. Place in bowl and toss together with parsley and watercress.

Add the vegetable oil of your choice (safflower seed oil, soybean oil, sunflower seed oil) as your first salad dressing. Add about three tablespoonsful of whatever oil you use. Now add the first of your seasonings. You can start with organic multiple mineral food substances if you like. This is a compound of finely ground vegetables and is usually sold in a container like a pepper shaker or bottle. It can be sprinkled directly onto the salad. Add one-half of a teaspoon of this seasoning to the ingredients. Toss all the greens in the bowl. Add one-half of a teaspoon of oregano. Toss all ingredients. You'll note at this point how well the oregano and mineral food substances cling to the oiled greens.

Dice one-third of a bunch of green onions (scallions). Add to salad. Dice one-third of a red onion. Add to salad. Toss all ingredients. Now add one or two teaspoonsful of lemon concentrate powder. Sprinkle on greens. Follow this by overlaying the lemon concentrate with the same quantity of orange concentrate powder. (These last two are optional, but I believe they add zest to the salad.) Toss ingredients again. Add a generous handful of alfalfa sprouts. Squeeze one-half of a fresh lemon onto salad. Toss ingredients. Add a tablespoonful of almond meal and toss.

Cut half a dozen Jerusalem artichokes into bitesize wedges. Add to salad. Cut either a dozen baby carrots or three large ones into thin slices. (Baby carrots are far superior in flavor.) Add to salad and toss ingredients. Slice thinly a medium-size wedge of red cabbage as if preparing for cole slaw. Add to salad.

Take one zucchini and one cucumber and cut up into quarter-inch segments. Add to salad and toss all ingredients. Now sprinkle enzyme powder freely on salad. Overlay this with another sprinkling of oregano and any or all of the other three powdered seasonings. Toss all ingredients again. Add one tablespoon of almond meal and toss again.

Chop into bitesize segments five to six stalks of green celery. Use the green parts of the celery, not the white, which are usually referred to as "hearts of celery." Add to salad. Now dice one-half of either a green or red pepper. Add to salad. Slice off the kernels of one or two ears of raw sweet corn. Add to salad and toss ingredients. Add one or two red ripe tomatoes. Cut into wedges and then slice wedges into quarters. Add to salad. (Be sure to add tomatoes last as they bruise easily and cannot take too much tossing.) Add juice of remaining half of lemon to salad. Toss ingredients, but lightly this time.

You now have a really superb vegetable salad, one that is properly prepared. You can, if you wish, replace the various oils and seasonings mentioned above with a French dressing rich in herbs. If you do, add a little of this dressing at a time as you prepare the salad—let us say after adding every third, fourth, or fifth vegetable to the bowl. Follow this by tossing ingredients evenly in bowl. In any case, avoid adding any salad dressing at the end of your preparations. You do not want the dressing to be concentrated on just a tiny portion of the salad. Otherwise, you will find it very flat to the taste.

At this point, you may eat the Alexander Salad as is or enrich it further with diced cheddar cheese, a can of tuna, or a pound of fresh shrimp, lobster, or crabmeat. You may, if you wish, add slices of leftover chicken. If you use the aforementioned seafoods, add a tablespoon of mayonnaise and toss all the ingredients one final time.

## SEVEN DAYS OF MENUS FOR THOSE WITH THINNING HAIR

### MONDAY

**BREAKFAST**
Alexander Hair Cocktail
(blended and taken as
described in Chapter 9)

**LUNCH**
½ canteloupe
Cottage cheese (1 cup)

**DINNER**
Alexander Salad (large
portion)
Steak (lean, 4 oz.)
Milk (8-oz. glass)

**OPTIONAL (10–11 P.M.)**
Wheat germ oil mixture
(mixed and taken as described in Chapter 9)

## TUESDAY

**BREAKFAST**
Alexander Hair Cocktail

**LUNCH**
Alexander Salad (small portion)
Broiled lean hamburger on wheat roll
Milk (8-oz. glass)

**DINNER**
Salmon steak, broiled (3 oz.)
Alexander Salad (large portion)
Strawberries and cream (or other berries in season)
Milk (10-oz. glass)

**OPTIONAL (10–11 P.M.)**
Wheat germ oil mixture

## WEDNESDAY

**BREAKFAST**
Alexander Hair Cocktail

**LUNCH**
Bowl of tomato and rice soup
Rye crackers and butter
Sliced orange (large)
Milk (8-oz. glass)

**DINNER**
Roast chicken (4 oz.)
Alexander Salad (large portion)
Ripe banana–sunflower seeds milk shake (use 8 oz. milk, 1 banana, and two tablespoonsful of sunflower seeds in blender)

**OPTIONAL (10–11 P.M.)**
Wheat germ oil mixture

## THURSDAY

**BREAKFAST**
Alexander Hair Cocktail

**LUNCH**
Fresh fruit salad
Yogurt—orange juice milk
shake (½ pint yogurt,
½ pint fresh orange
juice—no milk—mixed in
blender)

**DINNER**
Roast beef, medium rare
(4 oz.)
Alexander Salad (large
portion)
Choice of fruit
Milk (10-oz. glass)

**OPTIONAL (10–11 P.M.)**
Wheat germ oil mixture

## FRIDAY

**BREAKFAST**
Alexander Hair Cocktail

**LUNCH**
Tuna fish sandwich (use
whole-grain bread)
Grapefruit sections, fresh
(½ grapefruit)
Milk (10-oz. glass)

**DINNER**
Choice of soup
Whole-grain crackers
Butter (1 pat)
Choice of broiled fish or
meat (3 oz.)
Alexander Salad (medium
portion)
Milk or milk shake (no ice
cream—use yogurt, choice
of fruit and sunflower
seeds, plus almond meal)

**OPTIONAL (10–11 P.M.)**
Wheat germ oil mixture

### SATURDAY

**BREAKFAST**

Alexander Hair Cocktail

**LUNCH**

Hotdogs and beans
Pineapple wedges
Plain yogurt and sliced
banana
Milk (10-oz. glass)

**DINNER**

Broiled liver with onions
(6 oz.)
Alexander Salad (medium
portion)
Melon in season
Milk (10-oz. glass)

**OPTIONAL (10–11 P.M.)**

Wheat germ oil mixture

### SUNDAY

**BREAKFAST**

Alexander Hair Cocktail

**LUNCH**

Broiled lean hamburger on
wheat roll
Cole slaw
Choice of fruit
Milk shake (use plain
yogurt, orange juice, and
sunflower seeds in
blender)

**DINNER**

Large steak, broiled (4 oz.)
Alexander Salad (medium
portion)
Choice of soup
Choice of fruit
Milk (10-oz. glass)

**OPTIONAL (10–11 P.M.)**

Wheat germ oil mixture

## SEVEN DAYS OF MENUS FOR THOSE WITH
## VERY LITTLE HAIR

### MONDAY

**BREAKFAST**

Alexander Hair Cocktail
(enriched with 1 tbsp.
chia seeds—taken and
blended as described in
Chapter 9)

**LUNCH**

½ cup raw wheat germ
(served as a regular cold
cereal)
Sliced banana
Milk (10-oz. glass)

**DINNER**

Lentil soup (1 cup)
Roast beef, medium rare
(4 oz.)
Alfalfa sprouts–grated
carrot salad
*Fortified milk shake of
germinating seeds

**EVENING SNACK**

†chia seed pudding

---

* Blend 1 tsp. each of chia, sunflower, millet, pumpkin, and sesame seeds
with 8 oz. of milk.
† Blend raw milk, raw egg, and 1 tbsp. chia seeds. Refrigerate for two
hours, which allows gelatin from chia seeds to firm. A small piece of
papaya, or your favorite fruit, adds additional flavor.

## TUESDAY

BREAKFAST

Alexander Hair Cocktail
(enriched with 1 tbsp.
chia seeds)

LUNCH

Liver steak, medium rare
(½ lb.)
Raw, red onion (2–3 slices)
Baked potato
Butter (2 pats)
Green drink (use parsley,
watercress, and celery
blended with fresh pine-
apple and apple juice)

DINNER

Fresh salmon steak, broiled
(4 oz.)
Alexander Salad (large
portion)
Plain yogurt with fresh
fruit
Fortified milk shake of
germinating seeds

EVENING SNACK

Chia seed pudding

## WEDNESDAY

BREAKFAST

Alexander Hair Cocktail
(enriched with 1 tbsp.
chia seeds)

LUNCH

Bean soup (1 bowl)
Dark grain bread (1 slice—
use sprouted whole wheat
if available)
Butter (1 pat)
Minute steak, broiled
Sliced tomato
Milk (8-oz. glass)

DINNER

Lamb chops (lean), broiled
(4 oz.)
Baked potato
Butter (2 pats)
Alexander Salad (medium
portion)
Watermelon or choice of
melon
Fortified milk shake of ger-
minating seeds

EVENING SNACK

Chia seed pudding

### THURSDAY

**BREAKFAST**

Alexander Hair Cocktail
(enriched with 1 tbsp.
chia seeds)

**LUNCH**

Tuna fish and alfalfa
sprouts sandwich (use
sprouted whole wheat
bread if available)
Sliced orange and plain
yogurt
Milk (8-oz. glass)

**DINNER**

T-bone steak, broiled (4 oz.)
Alexander Salad (large
portion)
Cheese wedges
Fortified milk shake of
germinating seeds

**EVENING SNACK**

*Mixed nuts and raisins
(small portion)

* Mix equal parts of cashews, filberts, almonds, and macadamia nuts
with raisins. Use only unsalted, unroasted varieties of nuts generally
available at health food stores.

### FRIDAY

**BREAKFAST**

Alexander Hair Cocktail
(enriched with 1 tbsp.
chia seeds)

**LUNCH**

Bean and barley soup
(1 bowl)
Whole wheat crackers
Grapefruit sections
Plain yogurt and orange
juice milk shake

**DINNER**

Fish, meat, or fowl (4 oz.)
Choice of vegetable or fruit
salad
Whole wheat cooky
Fortified milk shake of
germinating seeds

**EVENING SNACK**

Chia seed pudding

## SATURDAY

**BREAKFAST**

Alexander Hair Cocktail
(enriched with 1 tbsp.
chia seeds)

**LUNCH**

Hamburger and alfalfa
sprouts sandwich
Green drink (use parsley,
watercress, and celery
blended with fresh pine-
apple or papaya and
apple juice)

**DINNER**

Filet mignon or choice of
steak, broiled (4 oz.)
Alexander Salad (large
portion)
Sliced orange and grape-
fruit sections
Fortified milk shake of
germinating seeds

**EVENING SNACK**

Cheese and choice of fruit

## SUNDAY

**BREAKFAST**

Alexander Hair Cocktail
(enriched with 1 tbsp.
chia seeds)

**LUNCH**

½ cup raw wheat germ
(serve as a regular cold
cereal)
Sliced banana
Mixed nuts (unsalted) and
raisins (add to cereal or
eat as a dessert—small
portion)
Milk (10-oz. glass)

**DINNER**

Roast beef, medium rare
(4 oz.)
Alexander Salad (large
portion)
½ canteloupe
Fortified milk shake of
germinating seeds

**EVENING SNACK**

Chia seed pudding

## SEVEN DAYS OF MENUS FOR THOSE WITH DANDRUFF PROBLEMS

### MONDAY

**BREAKFAST**
Alexander Hair Cocktail
(taken and blended as
described in Chapter 8)

**LUNCH**
Vegetable soup (1 bowl)
Broiled hamburger on
whole wheat bun
Sliced red onion
Milk (8-oz. glass)

**DINNER**
Shrimp cocktail
Steak or chops, broiled
Baked potato with chives
and sour cream
Alexander Salad (medium
portion)
Milk (8-oz. glass)

**10–11 P.M.**
*Vitamin-B milk shake

* Blend 8 oz. milk with 1 tbsp. each of brewer's yeast, desiccated liver, lecithin, raw wheat germ, and sunflower seeds. Choice of fruit (small piece) may be added for fruit flavor. Pineapple, apple, or banana recommended. Also add 1 tbsp. of either soybean oil or sunflower seed oil.

### TUESDAY

**BREAKFAST**
Alexander Hair Cocktail

**LUNCH**
Sunflower seed meal and
raw wheat germ mixed
(½ cup—serve as a
regular cold cereal)
Sliced banana
Milk (10-oz. glass)

**DINNER**
Calf's or beef liver, broiled
(6 oz.)
Red onion and red tomato
salad
Choice of melon in season
Milk (10-oz. glass)

**10–11 P.M.**
Vitamin-B milk shake

## WEDNESDAY

**BREAKFAST**

Alexander Hair Cocktail

**LUNCH**

Crabmeat, lobster, and
shrimp salad

Tomato and romaine
lettuce salad

Choice of raw fruit

Plain yogurt (8 oz.)

**DINNER**

Alexander Salad (medium
portion)

Roast beef, medium rare
(4 oz.)

Sliced orange

Milk (8-oz. glass)

**10–11 P.M.**

Vitamin-B milk shake

## THURSDAY

**BREAKFAST**

Alexander Hair Cocktail

**LUNCH**

Sunflower seed meal and
raw wheat germ mixed
(½ cup—serve as a
regular cold cereal)

Choice of fruit

Milk (8-oz. glass)

**DINNER**

Chicken or turkey, roasted
(4 oz.)

Baked potato with chives
and sour cream

Raw fruit

Plain yogurt (8 oz.)

Milk (8-oz. glass)

**10–11 P.M.**

Vitamin-B milk shake

### FRIDAY

**BREAKFAST**
Alexander Hair Cocktail

**LUNCH**
Raw fruit salad plate
Cheese wedges
Milk (8-oz. glass)

**DINNER**
Carrot juice (6-oz. glass)
Swordfish or halibut steak,
broiled (4 oz.)
Alexander Salad (medium
portion)
Cottage cheese and plain
yogurt
Milk (8-oz. glass)

**10–11 P.M.**
Vitamin-B milk shake

### SATURDAY

**BREAKFAST**
Alexander Hair Cocktail

**LUNCH**
Sunflower seed meal and
raw wheat germ mixed
(½ cup)
Sliced banana
Milk (8-oz. glass)

**DINNER**
Sirloin steak, broiled (4 oz.)
Baked potato with chives
and sour cream
Raw grapefruit sections
Cheese wedges
Milk (8-oz. glass)

**10–11 P.M.**
Vitamin-B milk shake

## SUNDAY

**BREAKFAST**

Alexander Hair Cocktail

**LUNCH**

Lentil soup (1 cup)

Hotdogs and beans

or

Cold cut meat plate and
beans

Plain yogurt and orange
juice milk shake

**DINNER**

Roast beef, medium rare
(4 oz.)

Alexander Salad (large
portion)

Choice of fresh fruit

Mixed nuts and raisins
(small portion)

Milk (8-oz. glass)

10–11 P.M.

Vitamin-B milk shake

## Special Points

1. Drink all the water you wish, but try to drink it
at least ten minutes before a meal or several hours
after it.

2. The same applies to coffee.

3. Use only saccharine or other sugar substitutes or
brown sugar in all instances where a sweet taste is
desired.

4. Use salt sparingly.

5. If you suffer from colitis or ulcers, to secure even
greater assurance that no irritation will occur use
larger amounts of oil when preparing the salad

than I have recommended. The oil will coat all the vegetables.

6. Avoid refined foods and all sweets and jellies unless made from natural products.

7. Remove fat from meats before broiling.

8. Take vitamin and food supplements at end of meals.

9. Use whole milk only. Stay away from nonfat or skimmed milk.

10. If you travel a lot and find the hair cocktail hard to manage, take along a bottle of raw wheat germ. Every morning, take half a cup of wheat germ and milk as your breakfast. Eat big portions of raw green salads at other meals. Remember always, even while you're traveling, that you are selecting your foods with an important goal in mind—the growth and health of your hair.

11. To replace nutrients that are lost in cooking, you may wish to add, as I do, various food supplements, vitamins, minerals, and digestive enzymes. I frequently add to my breakfast hair cocktail a tablespoonful of sunflower seed or soybean oil. I have also often added brewer's yeast, kelp powder, sunflower seed meal, calcium powder, and desiccated liver. These items can usually be found in health food stores.

In addition I take multiple vitamin-mineral capsules or tablets. These are made from natural products and are also available in health food stores.

(These supplements are not mandatory. But in my opinion, they will enrich the diet I have recommended and speed up the process of growing healthy hair.)

12. When yogurt is mentioned in the menus, plain yogurt only is meant.

# 11

## CONSTIPATION: IS IT A MENACE TO YOUR HAIR?

We have already noted how important diet is to hair health. The body receives its food by swallowing it. The physiologic counterpart of swallowing is defecation, the process by which the body rids itself of material from which it can no longer profit.

A constipated person loses his appetite and is apt to slight the proper diet. He may feel listless, apathetic, and will be uninterested in attempting to keep his scalp and his hair healthy and clean. In addition, there is no question that constipation gives some persons headaches. Whatever the mechanism by which headache occurs as a result of constipation, a headache usually means a change of circulation within the skull. This change of circulation is frequently reflected in changes of circulation in the arteries of the scalp, especially noticeable at the temples, where the arteries may throb vigorously and painfully. If chronic constipation leads to frequent headaches, which, in turn, lead to changes in the circulation of the scalp, it is conceivable that, in this indirect way, constipation could also contribute to baldness.

### Psychological Factors

Baldness can be thought of as, in part, psychosomatic, many cases having been reported where the hair has fallen out for psychological reasons, as the result of a sudden shock or overwhelming emotion. This is especially true of *alopecia areata,* described in a previous chapter. As for *alopecia seborrheica* and *alopecia prematura,* it is possible that small psychological traumas over a period of years in a susceptible scalp may lead to these diseases.

Like peptic ulcer or other psychosomatic diseases, the cure may be partly psychological and partly somatic —or bodily. For example, in spastic constipation, modern doctors not only attempt to persuade the patient to eat correctly and take the proper medications but they also try to point out his errors of thinking and behaving. Similarly, in baldness, while diet is the main consideration and hair cleanliness and scalp health of almost equal importance, it may also be necessary for the sufferer to change his mode of thinking and living to a more relaxed and low-pressured existence. Thus, he will digest his food better, get more nourishment from it, keep his occipitofrontalis muscles free from tension, and so allow better circulation to the scalp.

## The Colon

We may think of the large bowel, where constipation occurs, as the final reservoir of the gastrointestinal tract. Beyond being just a reservoir, it has several important functions. From the large bowel, or colon, the last bits of digested materials are absorbed into the circulation. The colon also withdraws certain substances from the blood and excretes them. Since digestion requires a fluid milieu, it can readily withdraw fluid from the bloodstream to provide this milieu.

The colon can be thought of as an incubator where certain helpful bacteria break down materials that have resisted previous digestive processes. The large bowel, or colon, churns and dehydrates the residue, returning to the circulation the all-important and life-giving fluid. These churning and pushing motions pack the residue, which we call feces or stool or bowel movement, into the rectum, the terminal portion of the large bowel. As the rectum distends and as more and more pressure builds up behind the sphincter muscle of the anus, we receive a signal in our brains that the wastes are ready to be disposed of.

We relax the sphincter and the "bowels move." This evacuation of residue is under nervous control and is a complex reflex act that may be hindered or helped by the contraction of certain voluntary muscles. If there is not sufficient fecal pressure built up to expel the remaining wastes, the person may make a conscious effort to build up sufficient pressure by closing the glottis (the opening between the vocal chords), holding the breath, and contracting the abdominal muscles, thus helping to force the wastes out.

## Spastic Colitis

When we think of the complexity of this physiology and the importance that people—particularly those of previous generations—put on regularity of bowel movement, we can understand what a major role the bowel plays in our lives. If we add to this the restrictions and inhibitions that have grown up about a perfectly normal function, common and necessary to all mankind, we arrive at an anatomical region and a mechanism second to none in its importance to our conscious and unconscious lives.

What frustrates a mother or father more than the child who fails in toilet training, especially bowel training? A Gesell Institute publication states: "Of all requests for help which we receive in the mail, letters asking for help in toilet-training problems are exceeded only by those asking for help with school problems." The psychologists, and most modern parents, understand that children will express anger or frustration by either refusing to defecate or doing it at an inappropriate time. This gives them "power" over the parent or nursemaid.

Some such mechanism may sometimes be carried over into adult life and appear as spastic colitis, characterized either by constipation or diarrhea. Bargen mentions overwork, overeating, insufficient rest, nervous fatigue, nervous tension, and exposure to the elements as among the immediate triggering causes of spastic colitis, or irritable bowel syndrome, as it is also known. Again, psychology is important.

There are other forms of constipation besides the irritable bowel syndrome. Any person who suffers from constipation should be examined by his physician to be sure there is no anatomical or pathological lesion that is causing it. If he has this reassurance, and if telling himself that the constipation is a form of resentment does not cure it, I believe he can cure himself in the same way *I* cured *myself*.

## Some Helps toward Regularity

I recommend this supplementary drink:

1. Eight ounces of milk heated to the point of being barely warm to the touch.
2. Two tablespoonsful of "raw" wheat germ.
3. One tablespoonful of flake-form brewer's yeast.
4. Two shredded, pitted prunes.

**5.** Two tablespoonsful of an unsaturated fat, such as soybean, sunflower seed, or safflower seed oil.

Blend thoroughly for one to two minutes in an electric blender. Taken at the close of a meal, it has done wonders for my constipation. It should be noted that this is a fine source of the B vitamin, as well as of the polyunsaturated oils. After regularity is reestablished, it may be taken as needed.

I offer a word of warning. Do not overdo the use of the above drink. Milk in excess quantities will cause gaseous distention in some susceptible individuals.

I also have found that yogurt—plain, no added attractions—and large quantities of uniced tap water are most helpful. Start the water when you arise, twenty to sixty minutes before breakfast, and keep it up at intervals all day, a glass at a time until six to ten glasses have been consumed.

If your constipation is atonic—that is, due to a lax colon—rather than spastic, the above-mentioned drink can be used, plus prunes, figs, and dates, taken in moderation. Excellent also are raw onions of any kind, salads made of raw vegetables, in particular the Alexander Salad (the recipe is given in another chapter), and raw fruits.

But again a word of warning. Sufferers from peptic ulcer or colitis of any kind may not do well on onions and raw vegetables, and should consult their physicians before embarking on this diet. Some persons tormented by ulcers will find that they can eat such a diet in the winter and summer but not in the spring or fall, when ulcers are apt to act up. They may also find that, when everything is going well, when life is just a bowl of cherries, they can eat said cherries, skin and all, and the aforementioned diet with impunity; but at other times they can eat almost nothing without suffering ulcer symptoms.

Yes, I believe that constipation *is* a menace to the hair and I believe that it is important for any balding person to watch his P's and Q's—Prunes and a Quota of raw vegetables. If constipation is a menace to the hair, let's do away with constipation.

# 12

## SHAMPOO AND MASSAGE: THEY FEEL FINE, BUT DO THEY DO ANY GOOD?

The beauty columns of newspapers and magazines are lavish with their advice on the care of the hair. How much of this advice is scientifically researched and how much is merely copied by one writer from another, is a question worth pursuing. Let me first give you some typical advice as culled from an assortment of women's magazines, and then allow me to comment on the validity of the suggestions.

### Dry Hair

If your hair is dry or has been parched by the sun, they urge you to use a cream conditioner. This, they claim, is good for both fine and coarse hair, giving the former more bulk and making the latter softer and easier to comb and set. Or they draw an analogy to a

151

piece of machinery, however erroneously: if your hair is dry, lubricate it with olive oil. Then comes advice on dull hair: shine it with an egg shampoo. Various ways of separating and combining the white and the yolk are given, but always the advice is to rub it in instead of swallowing it.

From a chemical point of view, of course, what is accomplished is to give bulk and stiffness to the hair with the albumen and to coat it with the fat of the yolk and thus make the hair shinier. No known nutritive value is contributed to the hair shaft or follicle as a result of rubbing them with any part of the egg. It makes a good deal more sense to *eat* the egg and let the bloodstream bring proteins and fats to the hair follicle where they are needed.

Eggs, preferably raw, fresh, and fertile, plus all the other good things listed in my diets, will do more to cure dry and dull hair than all the "conditioners" and egg shampoos. Remember, also, that hair is not a machine. It cannot be oiled successfully from the outside. It must be oiled from the bloodstream through the capillary tufts underlying each hair follicle and each sebaceous gland.

### Brushing

Then comes advice on brushing. Long, sweeping strokes are usually recommended. It is distinctly my impression that ladies with long hair are able to take that long stroke, while those with short hair must be content with a short stroke. "Brush from the scalp toward the ends," beauty columnists invariably say. Lady, just try brushing in the other direction with those long sweeping strokes. You'll end up with curly little bunches of "teased" hair, looking more like some aborigine than a modern housewife and mother!

The advice continues: "Brush 100 strokes (or 200 or 300)." I've figured out that it takes about one and one-half minutes to give a woman's hair 100 strokes of a brush, if she doesn't stop to rest; 300 strokes will take almost five minutes. Doesn't sound like much, but it would be an awful bore for most ladies to stand there and repeat the same motion for that length of time. The time would be more gainfully spent preparing an Alexander Salad.

Let us not forget the Eskimo. The early Eskimos had no hairbrushes; but they had beautiful, glistening heads of luxuriant jet-black hair, kept that way by a diet high in seal meat, whale blubber, and fish, all containing polyunsaturated fats. Now, don't get the idea that I'm against brushing the hair. I believe the hair should be brushed thoroughly every day. But forget the 100, 200, or 300 strokes. It should be obvious that people with long, thick hair will need to brush more than people with sparse hair. Those with coarse hair can afford to be less gentle than persons with fine hair.

Brush in the direction of the arterial circulation, then in the direction of the venous circulation, in order, first, to encourage a free flow of fresh blood to the scalp and, second, to hasten the removal of the wastes in the venous blood. I'm not proposing that you take a course in anatomy. Since the arteries and veins run, for the most part, side by side, just a few things need be remembered:

1. A line drawn from each side of the nape of the neck up the back of the head almost to the top marks the course of the occipital arteries and veins.

2. A line drawn from behind the earlobe to join the first line near the top of the head traces the course of the posterior auricular vessels.

3. A line drawn from the front of the earlobe to the junction of the first two lines traces the course of the superficial temporal vessels.

4. A line drawn from the top and front of the ear to the ridge above the eye traces the supraorbital vessels.

5. The small branches of all these vessels meet and join across the top of the scalp.

Therefore, when you brush, brush along the course of the arteries first, from the nape of the neck, from behind the ear, from in front of the ear, always toward the back of the crown and the middle of the crown, from the top of the front of the ear toward the front of the crown. After you have brushed briskly in these directions several times, reverse direction and brush from the crown toward the nape of the neck and the

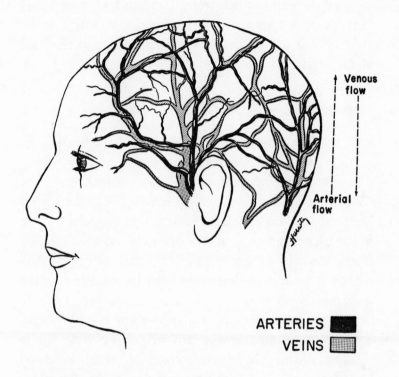

**Venous flow**

**Arterial flow**

ARTERIES ▮

VEINS ▨

## THE FINE ART OF HAIR BRUSHING

The above illustration, showing the circulatory system of the scalp, affords a guide to brushing the hair. Brush first in the direction of the arterial circulation, from the nape of the neck, from behind the ear, from in front of the ear toward the front of the crown. This will stimulate the flow of fresh nutritive blood to the capillary loops at the base of each hair. Then reverse the direction to flush "used" blood out of the capillary system.

back and front of the ear. Alternating these movements will help to flush fresh blood in and used blood out. It will be an aid in bringing the nutritive materials of your diet to the tiny capillary loops at the base of each hair.

## Massage

If brushing helps the circulation of the scalp, certainly massage will do at least as much. Lauder, Brunton, and others have shown that bloodflow through the tissues is actually increased by massage. Mitchell even believed that massage increased the hemoglobin value of the blood and the number of red blood cells and, by inference, the oxygen and nutritional supply to the tissues. A somewhat deeper and more vigorous massage is necessary to reach the arteries, which tend to lie deeper than the veins. So I suggest a few minutes twice a day of vigorous massage upward in the same directions as outlined in my section on brushing, followed by light, superficial massage in the opposite direction.

As an auxiliary to the proper diet, massage should not be ignored. In deeper massage, the scalp should be moved in the desired direction by the fingertips. This scalp movement is made possible by the layer of loose areolar tissue between the epicranium and the pericranium. In the more superficial massage, movement of the scalp is not necessary; gentle stroking motions will do. If your hair is very thick, be sure your fingers reach the scalp.

## Plucking

There is a technique to induce hair growth that is of great interest experimentally and seems to have some reference to our present problem. That is plucking. Starting with the experiments of Collins, as reported in the *Journal of Experimental Zoology* in 1918 and carried further by Herman B. Chase of Brown University, who wrote in *Physiological Reviews* in 1954, plucking of club hairs in resting follicles proved to be a most effective agent for initiating new hair growth from a resting follicle. Whether the club is plucked out or is broken off just above the follicle and then falls out by itself, the process acts as a stimulus to the new growth of hair in many experiments with animals and also in man.

Even vigorous grooming, short of breaking off or pulling out the hair, may have a similar effect in initiating a long anagen, or growth phase, and shortening the telogen, or resting phase, of the hair cycle. It is interesting that shaving or cutting, if the hair is not pulled, does not have this effect on the hair cycle; but depilatory agents, such as barium sulfide (used in many commercial hair removers for ladies' legs), do have a similar effect.

In *alopecia prematura* in man, the follicles have been found to have a very short growth phase. If some means could be found to change this short anagen phase back to a long anagen phase and do it quickly, efficiently, and steadily, I would be willing to concede that this would be a method even better than my diet. The latter takes considerable time and concentration, but at this moment is easily the best means available I know of. I see no practical application of plucking as a technique for stimulating hair growth in man in the foreseeable future.

## Shampooing

As far as shampooing goes, I'm all for it. I believe that, since the health of the hair derives from healthy blood and a healthy blood supply, hardly anything you might do from the outside can harm it. In a more positive vein, I believe that a clean scalp, free from excess sebum, which may cause alopecia, can more easily be kept in top-notch condition by the proper diet than a dirty scalp covered by sebum and scales.

You must shampoo your hair regularly. Don't worry about "drying the scalp" or "washing away the natural oils." You need not worry about insufficient oils while you are on my diet. Use a soapless shampoo, unless a dermatologist tells you specifically that you are being harmed by this type of shampoo, which is highly unlikely. As far as antidandruff shampoos are concerned, I believe that a soapless shampoo used often enough will keep dandruff under control as effectively as a dandruff-removing or dandruff-"curing" shampoo. These "cures" usually contain either sulfur, which smells awful and will turn black in the sunlight if it isn't washed out thoroughly with another shampoo, or selenium, which is known to cause hair thinning in some susceptible persons. Selenium is poisonous if taken internally, so one must be careful to keep it out of the reach of children.

Since shampoos containing selenium tend to deteriorate if subjected to heat or light, they are usually marketed in opaque bottles liberally sprinkled with warnings. Shampoos containing tar seem harmless except to those allergic to them; but the odor reminds me of a dog being treated for mange, and I find that particular fragrance hard to take. Another caution—shampoos containing sulfur may discolor silver jewelry or other metal objects and may even stain your sink or wall permanently.

Don't forget that dull hair may represent nothing more than a film left on the hair by a precipitate from hard water. This can be avoided by using distilled water or rain water, or by adding a teaspoonful of bicarbonate of soda, better known as baking soda, to the rinse water, if you live in a district that derives its water from a hard-water source, such as an artesian well.

## Ladies, Beware!

Some warnings for the ladies:

1. Avoid nylon bristles unless your hair is very thick and needs to be thinned; even then, it is best to let a professional hairdresser thin your hair systematically rather than cut it with a nylon-bristled brush.

2. Check your comb when you buy it to make sure it has no rough tips that may cut your hair or entangle it and drag it out of your scalp.

3. Avoid metal curlers with sharp edges.

4. Avoid brush-type rollers or any other type of roller that may put too much tension on your hair.

5. Don't stick to one hair style too long; with today's bouffant and sculptured hairdos, too much tension on any one area of the scalp for too long may result in "tension alopecia."

6. When setting or rolling your hair, allow enough slack between the roller and the scalp to avoid undue tension; don't forget that there is a slight shrinkage of the hair, as there is in almost any natural fiber, between the wet and the dry state.

7. Even if you wind the hair loosely and leave enough slack, you may provoke too much tension by sleeping in your rollers; either do your hair early enough in the day or use a hair dryer to avoid sleeping with a head full of porcupines. If you are afraid of losing the set, tie each curl in place with toilet tissue or, more glamorously, some colorful ribbon; you can cover the whole thing with an attractive cap or net.

8. And last, a personal warning: I've found out through talking to men around the country that a lot of men are really fed up with you gals in rollers —at work, in the street, in bed. Take 'em off!

# 13

# WIGS, TOUPEES, HAIRPIECES, AND HAIR WEAVING: IF YOU CAN'T GROW, SEW!

If you have been *completely* bald for more than five years, I'm afraid that my methods won't do you any good. For the benefit of my own friends who were suffering from this sad condition, I gathered what material I could on the periwig, or wig as it is now known. I offer it here for those of you who have been long hairless or who have an interested friend or relative in that predicament.

While the wig is usually worn to conceal baldness, or to conceal what the wearer considers inadequate hair, it may also be part of a professional, ceremonial, fashionable, or stage costume. Judges and barristers in England, medicine men and tribal dancers, models and fashionable ladies, actors and actresses the world over have worn them—even when not bald. Thus the wig can be an adornment, a disguise, or a symbol of office.

## History of Wigs

Wigs are of such great antiquity that they have been found on Egyptian mummies. There is some evidence that the Egyptian ladies, being dark haired, naturally wanted to be blondes. So they put lye and potash on their heads and sat in the sun to bleach their hair. This probably burned their scalps, made their hair brittle, and thinned it out. To cover the damage, as well as to change their styling, they adopted wigs. The Egyptian women were also known for the use of that perennial favorite, henna, which turns the hair red.

In ancient Greece, both men and women wore wigs, while both Xenophon and Aristotle mention that wigs were worn by the Medes and the Persians. Greek actors were apt to adorn their theatrical masks with black hair to represent a tyrant, blond curls for a hero, and red hair for the dishonest slave who was a popular comic figure, as was the redheaded stage Irishman in the early days of our own theater.

In Rome, upperclass ladies of fashion loved wearing false hair, as do similar groups in our own day. The Roman ladies especially favored golden locks imported from what we now call Germany, and the notorious Empress Messalina wore a blond wig for her visits to the local bordellos. The Empress Faustina had several hundred wigs in her wardrobe. So popular was the wig that portrait-bust statues have been found in which the hair was removable and could be replaced by any hair fashion current at the moment. The Louvre has such a bust, but I don't know if they are still changing the wig to keep the statue *au courant*. It seems to me a trust they shouldn't shirk!

In seventeenth-century France, the wig, or peruke, became a feature of the fashionable costume, since Louis XIII was bald himself and wore a peruke to conceal this shortcoming; the fashion spread throughout Europe from the court of Versailles. In England, under Charles II, the wearing of wigs became almost universal, at least among those who could afford them. Under Queen Anne, the wig became so highly developed that it covered the back, shoulders, and chest. Wigs became differentiated according to class in society and according to profession, which accounts for their persistent popularity through the ages with doctors, lawyers, clergymen, and soldiers. Today, only Great Britain still clings to the wig as official dress; they are still worn there by the speaker of the House of Commons, the clerks of Parliament, the Lord Chancellor, and judges and barristers.

## Theatrical Hairpieces

Early theatrical wigs of the European and American stage were constructed of any available material that resembled human hair. The wool of the sheep, the hair of goats, yaks, and horses, even jute fibers were used. Scarce llama hair was adopted for white wigs. It didn't matter too much what was used, since stage lighting depended on candles at first and oil lamps later. In the general gloom, the details of hair could certainly not be seen.

As lighting improved, so did wigs, and human hair came into general use. Modern theatrical wigs are sewn hair-by-hair through a soft gauze, and made to order for a particular actor or actress playing a particular character. The beautiful red wig that Gertrude Lawrence wore in *The King and I* on the Broadway musical stage was a masterpiece of the modern wig-maker's art and added glamour to her stage appearance. It contrasted markedly with the completely bald head of her leading man, Yul Brynner, who made a name for himself not only through fine acting but through his courage in appearing completely bald before millions of viewers via stage, screen, and television.

## Widening Uses of Wigs

Today, the techniques laboriously worked out over many years by theatrical wig-makers are being applied to nontheatrical wigs used by the society queen or the queen of the secretarial pool. At almost any price, wigs of imported human hair, small hairpieces on combs or on hairpins, imitation wiglets constructed from man-made fibers, wigs in every color, including some that never appeared in God-made hair, are available in beauty shops, drugstores, and even variety stores.

Nearly as widely available are wigs, toupees, and hairpieces for men. Varying in size from full Beatle mops through the toupee, which covers the bald top of the head and blends with the normal sides and back of the scalp hair, to the small hairpieces with which a matinee idol can fill in a receding hairline, they are used not only professionally but by countless thousands of men in their daily lives. Available in all natural colors, the wigs often defy detection except on close inspection or under unusual circumstances that cause them to go awry. Witness the old Irish expression, "wigs on the green," referring to a good fight when wigs were apt to fall on the grass.

Why this revival in modern dress of an old custom? Obviously, a wig or hairpiece can help a balding man attain a better job, a more positive personality, perhaps even a more successful love life. It is a well-known fact that the more satisfied we are with our appearance, the more general assertiveness we display. This self-confidence radiates outward and impresses prospective employers or customers. More poise, more assurance, improved performance on the job have resulted in increased income and positions entailing increased responsibility.

## Modern Technological Advances

Let's now drop consideration of all hairpieces and wigs except those used by the ordinary, everyday person, man or woman, to hide varying degrees of baldness. Before the Second World War, hair from Asia, chiefly China, was used in these wigs. The demand was not too great, and the supply seemed almost unlimited; so the price was within the reach of almost everyone. As a result of the Japanese takeover in Manchuria in 1936, and later the cessation of American trade with Communist China, our largest source of human hair was lost.

We then began to obtain hair from European sources that had less abundant supplies. The price of hair began to mount. Our own chemists then produced manmade fibers, such as Dynel, which make an excellent substitute for human hair, unless it is examined closely by a relatively expert eye. The use of artificial fibers now enables almost any woman to wear elaborate hairdos, pieced out and puffed out with inexpensive "hair'" pieces. Artificial fibers are also used with less satisfactory results in some low-priced toupees for men.

## Wefting and Joining

The following information was obtained from a series of interesting conversations with wig authority Martin Krever, one of New York's leading experts on hair styling. According to Krever, there are two major methods for making wigs and hairpieces nowadays. The first method is termed "wefting and joining." This is crude, quick, relatively inexpensive; and it enables the wig-maker to use hair of nonuniform length. A fringe is created by braiding string, artificial fibers, or hair at one end. The fringe is sewn onto tape. A ponytail or braid is then made from short pieces held in the

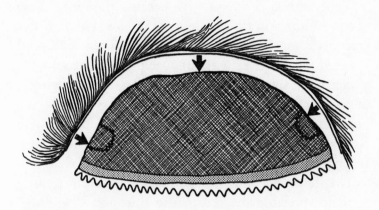

## WEFTING AND JOINING—ONE APPROACH
## TO THE PROBLEM

In this relatively inexpensive process for making wigs, the hairs are
sewn to a base of net or wired into a wire mesh to form a wig. A serious drawback to this method is that the hair tends to drift back to the
position into which it was originally sewn.

center strand by the central, concealed braid. When the fringes are laid one upon the other and sewn to a base of net or wired onto a wire mesh in a spiral effect, a wig is formed.

This method is inexpensive because the maker does not need uniform or long lengths of hair. He need not treat each hair individually, so the method is fast. And he need not be careful about spacing the hair equally, which again speeds up the wig-making. The drawbacks of this method are manifold. Since the hair is pre-positioned and directioned, styling must be limited. Regardless of how it is set by the hairdresser or wearer, it tends to drift back to the position into which it was originally sewn. The effects obtained are clumsy, since it is not possible to control the thickness. "Joining" refers to the formation of a ponytail, braid, chignon, or figure eight by attaching lengths of hair together end-to-end.

### Hand-Venting

The best method of wig-making is "hand-venting." In this method, carefully chosen hairs of the proper length are knotted individually through silk netting. By filling in or skipping some space, the weight and thickness of the wig can be controlled precisely. The hair can be set in any direction and tends to stay where set. It can even be parted successfully, if the netting used at the part is flesh-colored. It is the closest method

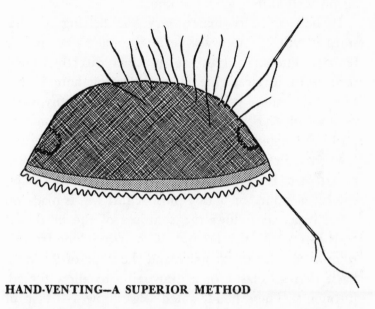

## HAND-VENTING—A SUPERIOR METHOD

Although the hand-venting method is more expensive than the weft-ing and joining method of wig construction, it is far superior. This process comes closest to simulating natural hair, and the wig may even be parted. There is one serious disadvantage, however; since the wig must be glued to the scalp, it can be used on totally bald areas only.

yet devised to natural hair that grows from a flesh-and-blood scalp. Silk seems to be the most durable of all fibers for the netting; and it resists perspiration damage as well as damage by sebum.

In hairpieces for males, very fine netting is used, since it will be more visible in the male than in the female. The hairpieces are attached directly to the scalp with surgical glue. The limitation here is that the pieces can be used on *totally bald areas only,* since removal of a hairpiece glued on with surgical glue will pull out whatever hair remains.

For females, a more substantial net is used. The wig or hairpiece is attached to the normal hair with clamps, combs, hairpins, or bobby pins. A full wig is made on a net cap that follows the contours of the head and ends just a half-inch behind the hairline. The front is reinforced with metal strips and the nape of the neck has either an elastic or a drawstring to allow for adjustments. These hand-vented wigs allow a stream of air to flow through and so are cooler and better protected from perspiration damage.

For any suspicious characters among my readers, let me say that all hair is first wound on metal rods, then boiled in water and sterilized before it is fashioned into anything. This process of boiling also makes it wavy and more manageable. Please note also that a wig or a hairpiece can be bleached, dyed, or waved in the same manner as your own hair. Prolonged use of wigs or hairpieces seems to have no adverse effect on the natural hair or scalp, unless there is prolonged pressure or tension in one spot. If this takes place, tension baldness will occur at that spot.

## Hair Weaving

Rapidly coming into popularity in recent years is the technique of hair weaving, which many now consider the next best thing to growing your own crop. Actually hair weaving, or hair sewing, has been utilized for many years by Negro beauticians for clients who want to achieve the appearance of long straight hair but do not want to resort to the usual hair-straightening techniques. It has recently been popularized by humans of both sexes and both colors, but mostly by the white male, as an alternative to, and in many respects an improvement over, the toupee.

Hair weaving can only be utilized if there is a base of existing hair to work with. Nylon threads are interwoven, close to the scalp, with the existing hair to form a meshwork base. To this base hanks of human hair, obtained from the usual markets in Europe and elsewhere, are sewn. These hanks can be mingled with one's own hair in such a way as to cover the bald areas. The effect, if the job is competently done, is that of a healthy-looking head of hair.

Since the added hair is not attached to the scalp with glue or tapes, as with a toupee, the individual can be more carefree about diving into a swimming pool or participating in other activities. The chief disadvantage is that, since the natural hair continues to grow, the hanks of hair attached to it will also move away from the scalp—but without reinforcements from below as with one's own hair, thus creating a credibility gap. This means that the hanks must be unwoven and rewoven at fairly frequent intervals, usually every two or three months.

Another disadvantage is that this relatively new procedure—as far as its wide general application is concerned—has attracted many unskilled operators who seek to cash in on the trend. It is a highly specialized technique, one that is not effectively applied by the average beautician without extensive training, and it would be well if only licensed operators were permitted to practice hair weaving. Until then, it is very much a case of let the buyer of hair beware.

If it is too late for you to regrow your own hair, or if you haven't the willpower to follow the regimen I outline—and it does require plenty of willpower—take advantage of the skilled wig-maker's or hair-weaver's art. But if there is still a chance for you to till your own field, I urge you to try it.

# 14

# THE SURGICAL TREATMENT OF BALDNESS: SOME CUTTING REMARKS

Starting with the early Arabian physicians and continuing through the medieval Italians, skin grafting has evolved into a highly complicated and technically involved science. Its early history shows that it was popular in countries where cutting off of the nose was used as a punishment for various crimes. The victim, understandably, was willing to go through torture in order to get this most prominent feature replaced. And torture it was, since the early techniques involved a graft from the arm to the nasal area while the arm was tied tightly to the head for many days until the graft "took." The lack of suitable anesthesia, or even effective sedatives, added to the horror of the procedure and testify to the desperation of any patient who undertook this operation.

The great British and French surgeons of the time of the First World War made fantastic advances in skin grafting and laid down the principles that still are the basis of our present operations. But they were concerned with important injuries and didn't have the time or the interest to consider skin grafts for baldness. After the Second World War, interest in cosmetic plastic surgery grew. Noses were reshaped, faces pulled taut, baggy eyelids made young again; even breasts could be ordered in any desired size.

But no one, until recently, seemed to have any great interest in helping the poor bald man.

## A Variety of Recent Grafting Techniques

Many techniques have now been introduced, all still more or less on an experimental basis.

Interestingly enough, surgeons in Japan, where baldness is less of a problem than it is in the West, have transplanted *individual hairs* into bald areas, with some temporary success. In the United States, a surgeon named Foster has anchored nylon thread to nylon arrowheads and implanted the latter in the scalp through a hypodermic needle. He reports that nylon is fifteen times stronger than human hair, and that it can be made even stronger by irradiating it. He emphasizes that the nylon must be of uniform diameter throughout or it will break at a thin spot. Doctors are eagerly waiting to hear more of this method, especially bald doctors.

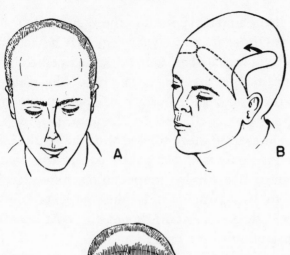

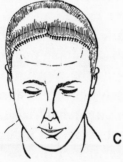

## THE LAMONT METHOD OF HAIR GRAFTING

This method of grafting, first reported in 1957, requires the taking of flaps of skin attached at one end, called *Pedicle Grafts,* from the temple area on each side of the scalp and sewing them across the former hairline in the front.

- *A.* The bald area.
- *B.* Illustration shows how flap is taken from the temple area and drawn across the former hairline.
- *C.* The appearance of hair six months after the operation.

In 1957, Lamont reported in the *Western Journal of Surgery, Obstetrics and Gynecology* that he had taken flaps of skin attached at one end, called pedicle grafts, from the temple area on each side of the scalp and sewed them across the former hairline in the front. The grafts grew well, and Dr. Lamont, judging from his article, seemed quite pleased with the result. I must say, judging only from the published pictures, that the result looks like a living toupee to me. What has happened to this patient and other patients similarly treated in the years since, I do not know. At least there is no mortality to the operation.

Iturrospe and Arufe, in Buenos Aires, used a multiplicity of procedures. A simple one to reduce the size of the bald scalp pulls the remaining edges together. This, of course, did not grow any new hair, but it brought the remaining hair edges closer together and made the victim *seem* less bald. They also used several different types of grafting techniques to move hairy sections to bald areas.

### Transplantation

Dr. Norman Orentreich did what was perhaps the most scientific and complete work on grafting for baldness. He reported this work in the *Annals* of the distinguished New York Academy of Sciences in 1959. He made grafts the full thickness of the scalp with a biopsy punch, the grafts being round and varying in diameter from six to twelve millimeters. He made sure

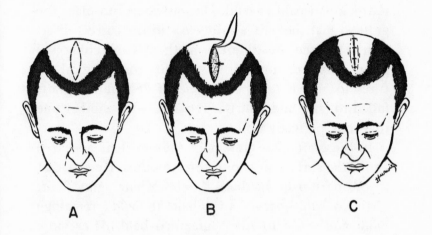

A        B        C

## THE ITURROSPE AND ARUFE
## METHOD OF HAIR RESTORATION

With this method Doctors Oturrospe and Arufe reduced the size of the bald area by removing an entire section of the bald scalp and pulling the remaining edges together. This method does not grow any new hair, but it makes one *seem* less bald.

*A.* Area of the scalp to be removed.
*B.* Flap of scalp is entirely removed.
*C.* Scalp is sewn together, thus reducing the bald area.

that he was below the hair follicles. Taking the grafts from normal scalp and from bald scalp, he then transplanted normal to normal, normal to bald, bald to normal, and bald to bald. He was careful to place the graft so that the hair would grow in the correct direction. He used six different methods of keeping the grafts in place, running the gamut from surgical sutures to Scotch tape. Only one of 284 punch grafts failed to take, and that was replaced with another one that took perfectly well.

In the grafts that grew hair, the new hair appeared above the surface in two to three months. He says that in ordinary male baldness, "hair to hair" grew hair; "hair to bald" grew hair; "bald to bald" remained bald; and "bald to hair" remained bald. After more than two years of observation, the graft continued to grow the same kind of hair that was present on it before it was transplanted. When the grafts were placed at a receding hairline, the patient's own hairline continued to recede behind the front graft; but the hair of the graft grew well. In other types of alopecia, the results were not nearly so spectacular.

In recent years this technique has become more widely accepted. Applying Dr. Orentreich's biopsy punch, dermatologists have performed this grafting technique on more than 5,000 American men. The relatively small number of operations is due in large measure to the cost. The cost of each graft is at present about $5. Considering that an estimated 200 such grafts

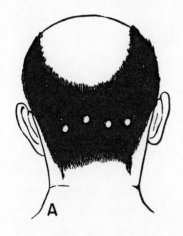
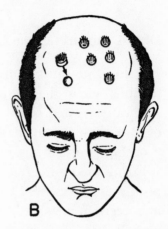

# HAIR TRANSPLANTATION

Perhaps the most successful of the various types of skin grafting was devised by Dr. Norman Orentreich in 1959. Using a biopsy punch, Dr. Orentreich removes a graft, or plug, the full thickness of the scalp from an area of the head on which normal hair grows. Making sure that he is below the hair follicle, he then transplants this plug into a bald area, taking care to place the graft so that the hair will grow in the correct direction. Grafts continue to grow the same kind of hair that was present before transplantation and in two to three months new hair begins to appear above the surface of the scalp.

*A.* Grafts or plugs are removed from an area of normal hair growth.

*B.* Grafts are then implanted in the bald area. They continue to grow normal hair despite transplantation.

might be needed to correct the average case of male pattern baldness, the total treatment often comes to $1,000.

## Diet vs. Surgery—Some Conclusions

I think we must admit that surgery for baldness is feasible, but in the not-too-near future. I feel that the surgically treated scalp will not have the appearance of a normal, nonbald scalp. Perhaps something approaching normality can be achieved by the most skillful of dermatosurgeons; but even in their hands the results, as represented by the pictures in medical journals, seem to me a little freakish. It reminds me of the man I once saw who covered his entirely bald scalp with a very thin layer of vaseline and then sprinkled it with hair shavings. He didn't look bald, but he didn't look normal, either.

Now, what are the advantages and disadvantages of surgical methods as compared to dietary therapy? Surgery offers "instant hair"; that is, the wound heals in a week, and the hair begins to appear in two to three months. With dietary therapy, it takes several months for the NuGrow Cycle to manifest itself. With surgery, any area of the scalp can be treated; with diet, only the hair lost in the last five years will be regrown. However, with surgery one does not know which graft will take and which won't. It is painful and takes you out of circulation for a period of time, unless you care to go to work with a turban over your wounds.

In any surgery, there is always the chance of infection and the chance of allergic reaction to the drugs used for anesthesia. While the scalp, because of its excellent blood supply, does not become infected easily, when it does become infected the infection can spread quickly and widely through the lax areolar tissue between the epicranium and the pericranium. If the hair receded all around a graft, the latter would take on the appearance of a hairy wart and the victim would probably insist upon having it removed. And I maintain that, if you do not nourish these grafted areas correctly with the hair cocktail and the diet I outline, they may "wither on the vine." If you were to grow hair by meticulous attention to the dietary recommendations I make, it would not look like a toupee; it would look normal because it would *be* normal.

At this time, skin can only be grafted from a person to himself, or from one identical twin to another. Experiments now being conducted are attempting to graft skin from any person to another, or from another animal to man. So far, the only near-successes have involved the use of dangerous chemicals or even more dangerous irradiation to knock out the mechanisms that reject grafts. I hope these experiments succeed. I have my eye on a particularly beautiful silken-haired chimp in the local zoo who could make a luxuriant contribution to my scalp.

# 15

## QUESTIONS ONE HEARS MOST ABOUT HAIR— AND THE ANSWERS

My first book, *Arthritis and Common Sense,* was published in three different hardcover editions. After the first edition was issued, I started out on a lengthy lecture tour. The questions I was asked during this tour convinced me that the book's language was too abstruse to be grasped by everyone who read it. So I did a great deal of clarifying and elucidating in a second edition published a year later.

Then I found that the print in the book was too small for the "age level" of the eyes that were attracted to the book. In dealing with the subject of arthritis, I was naturally reaching more older people—people with a preference for larger print. In addition to having the book reset in larger type, I added a chapter on the questions most frequently asked during my lectures on arthritis.

When I saw that it was possible for me to regrow hair, as well as control thinning hair and stop dandruff in its tracks, I decided to deliver a few lectures before the book on hair was written. I wanted above all to find out what my *public* wanted to know. In other words, what I wanted to do then, and what I believe I have accomplished in this book, is to publish the "third" edition first.

I began my series of lectures in Southern California. I lectured in my favorite city first, the very city where I began my eleven-year lecture tour on *Arthritis and Common Sense*—in beautiful Santa Monica. The first major lecture for the purpose of collecting questions on hair growth from an audience was delivered Wednesday, March 6, 1963, at the McKinley School Auditorium. It was sponsored by the Santa Monica Organic Garden and Nutrition Club. The audience was remarkably responsive. They definitely wanted to know more about the relationship between hair and diet. They sent their questions up to the platform.

The same thing happened with my audiences in Hollywood. There were four lectures in Hollywood. Then there were three lectures in Beverly Hills, one of them before the distinguished Saints and Sinners Club, a group of 200 people, at the Beverly Hilton Hotel. A lecture was also held at the Women's Club in Palm Springs. Some very keen questions were asked by both men and women. Then I spoke before the Senior Citizens' group. The next day, in Riverside, I addressed another group interested in healthy hair.

Everywhere, I invited the questions that, when answered, would help make this book the best available on the subject.

In this chapter I will answer these questions on hair. I will also include some questions that were asked about scalp and skin and nails, since they are all interrelated. The answers come from my own long years of search for the answers to health through nutrition and hygiene.

Perhaps the list of questions that follows will stimulate you into taking action about your own diet and other habit patterns. They may be the very questions that have long puzzled you about your own hair. One key question, answered correctly, may alone make this book the best investment you ever made. It may help to lift a cloud of indecision and thus spur you to action at last. These questions, for the most part, would almost certainly be the ones you would ask me if we ever had the pleasure of meeting personally.

Who knows—someday we may meet. I lecture in almost every section of the country. And I do not confine my activities to the United States. Not long ago I lectured extensively throughout South Africa, Australia, and New Zealand before the staffs of their medical universities, as well as before the general public. When I appeared on *Meet the Press* in Sydney, Australia, the leading doctors fired their sharpest questions at me through the top newspaper editors of Australia. I love to exchange knowledge with people. It's a salutary way to gain experience.

If I have already visited your city, I may be back again. Quite often the interest shown in one of my lectures has brought me back to give a second or third lecture in the same auditorium. Perhaps a relative or friend of yours has already attended one of my lectures.

Here, then, are *your* questions answered—a selection of the queries I hear most often.

**1.** QUESTION: How many eggs are you supposed to consume in one day to encourage hair growth?

ANSWER: Actually, one egg is sufficient. Whatever the number, they should preferably be fertile eggs and they must be raw. If fertile eggs are not available, regularly available eggs will do. They can be beautifully blended in a blender. To the eggs you add a selected group of germinating oils and food supplements. It is a balanced mixture of different products designed to meet different goals of the hair-growing program. Growing hair is a technique and it must be practiced diligently and faithfully.

**2.** QUESTION: Is it okay to boil the fertile eggs?

ANSWER: No. Boiling destroys the fertility the hair needs.

**3.** QUESTION: What causes a tight scalp?

ANSWER: Primarily the loss of the fatty layer of the scalp. It signifies the absence of hair follicles and skin atrophy.

4. QUESTION: How does one get rid of dandruff?

ANSWER: Dandruff is a difficult problem to overcome. The best way to attack the condition is to get professional hair care at a hair specialist's office. The hair must be thoroughly cleansed with properly selected solutions. Proper stimulation should be started through a scalp massaging program. Hairbrushing, effectively carried out, will accomplish wonders. Then, simultaneously, while a hair hygiene program is being carried out, the diet that is causing the scalp to form dandruff must be thoroughly regulated. New foods must be incorporated into the daily diet to nourish the scalp and hair, as explained in detail in the earlier chapters on this subject.

5. QUESTION: Why does hair fall only in the autumn of the year?

ANSWER: This is a fallacy. Hair may seem to fall more in the autumn. If, after a hot summer season, your hair is suffering from the effects of too much ice cream, too many soft drinks, too many candy-coated foods and similar snacks, it will thin noticeably. Hair will not flourish under this kind of nutritional punishment. Several weeks of foods loaded with sugar will contribute to falling hair.

**6.** QUESTION: What should one do about excessively oily hair?

ANSWER: Eliminate the wrong oils from the diet, such as ice cream, chocolate, bacon, or any oil, good or bad, that has been heated to a high temperature.

**7.** QUESTION: What causes baldness?

ANSWER: The absence of germinating foods in the diet, the presence of wrong foods like ice cream and soft drinks in the diet, a failure to keep the scalp and hair meticulously clean, the use of the wrong types of film-producing soaps, the failure to stimulate the scalp—and a host of other reasons you can dig out of this book.

**8.** QUESTION: Does Zone Therapy help the hair?

ANSWER: I don't see how this limited measure could benefit hair.

**9.** QUESTION: What harm does hair dye do to your hair?

ANSWER: Little by little, in my belief, dyes sap its strength. How do I know? I don't.

It is my educated guess. I also believe that if your diet is faulty, hair dyes are even more harmful to the hair.

**10. QUESTION:** What is your opinion of the wig craze?

**ANSWER:** Crazy, man, crazy. Each to her own taste. Personally, I prefer a girl who stands on her own hair. However, if a man is completely bald, a wig or surgical transplantation is his only resort.

**11. QUESTION:** What foods do you recommend to help restore color to the hair?

**ANSWER:** As a key food, I suggest brewer's yeast in flake form and other products rich in B-complex. Calcium pantothenate, part of the vitamin B complex, has been known to restore color to gray hair.

**12. QUESTION:** What can be done for dry skin and hair?

**ANSWER:** Including both hair and skin in the same question is completely logical. Anything that affects one affects the other. The best way to correct dry hair is to follow the rules in Chapter Twelve and the rules of diet stated throughout the book apply to both hair and skin.

**13. QUESTION:** How does one overcome patchy baldness?

ANSWER: If you are referring to *alopecia areata,* see Chapter Six.

**14.** QUESTION: What makes scaly skin form at the hairline?

ANSWER: It can be a sign of seborrhea, of a psychological skin disease called neurodermatitis, or of many other skin disorders.

**15.** QUESTION: What shampoo do you recommend?

ANSWER: The best grade of soapless shampoo. It must be soapless.

**16.** QUESTION: What do you recommend for falling hair?

ANSWER: About a hundred different things—mostly found in this book. The key is germinating foods.

**17.** QUESTION: I've heard that, if you can stand the smell, the following formula will grow hair: equal parts of flower of sulfur, oil of tar, and linseed oil.

ANSWER: Sounds like a great formula for a tractor—not for the scalp.

**18.** QUESTION: How do you overcome excessive dryness of the skin?

ANSWER: See Question 12.

**19.** QUESTION: What do you recommend to rid the scalp of oil, dead skin, so that the hair can come back to normal?

ANSWER: If there is more than 25 percent loss of hair, it is recommended that skin-peeling be done by professional hair specialists. Others will profit most from daily shampooing plus proper hair stimulation and bodily exercise.

20. QUESTION: What foods will prevent hair from turning gray?

ANSWER: No foods that I know of can actually by themselves prevent gray hair. Foods rich in vitamin B-complex may aid in the delay of hair color change.

21. QUESTION: What do you recommend for teen-ager's acne?

ANSWER: No fried foods, including potato chips. These foods contain a great deal of fats that may overload the oil glands whose openings become plugged in acne. The acne sufferer must not eat chocolate, ice cream, candy, soft drinks, and similar sweets, because his skin particularly is unable to handle an increased amount of sweets, and the oil glands become overactive and irritated.

22. QUESTION: If your program for regrowing hair is so good, why are you still partially bald?

ANSWER: I will never have a full head of hair. All I hope to recover is the hair I have lost in the past five years. It is my hope that I can continue to regenerate the fuzz areas where dying follicles still exist. I have been partially bald or balding since I was sixteen. It is not important that I regrow all my hair. What is important is that I, and anyone else afflicted with the same problem, stop losing the hair we have and attempt to regrow some of the hair we lost through a sensible diet program accompanied by proper hair cleansing, massage, and brushing.

**23. QUESTION:** I know a Mormon schoolteacher, a champion tennis player, who is almost completely bald—hair only around the sides of his head. He is in his twenties and very religious, does not smoke or drink. He did not harm his hair enzymes by indulging in soft drinks or candy. Why is he bald?

**ANSWER:** In all probability he didn't eat germinating foods. These foods are a must. The lowly onion, for example, is an extremely valuable germinating food. Yet entire families often never see a raw organic onion on the table, let alone a hair-nourishing salad. Other families serve the onion "cooked to death." For even the lowly onion to help germinate your hair, it must be served raw and it must be a fresh onion, not stale. And aside from diet, there are people who, because of hereditary and other causes, are doomed to baldness at an early age.

**24.** QUESTION: How does one correct an itching scalp? I try to eat properly—mostly health foods.

ANSWER: You are probably making the classic mistake so many health food followers make. You give up white sugar, ice cream, chocolate, soft drinks, and the like. You then proceed to buy honey, organic ice cream, carob, dietetic soft drinks, and the like. You get the point. You are merely swapping white sugar for brown sugar. If you have an itchy scalp, you cannot introduce even brown sugar for at least a year. Honey, dried fruits, and the like are loaded with concentrated sugar. They may be used, yes, but in moderation only.

**25.** QUESTION: What can be done about excessive dandruff? Should I shampoo my scalp more frequently?

ANSWER: Stop the sweets—both white sugar and brown sugar and the honey and the

sun-dried fruits. Add vital vegetable oils
to your diet. What kind of shampoo are
you using? Make sure it is a soapless
shampoo. We do not want to leave any
soap film. Shampoo daily.

**26. QUESTION:** What food would you recommend for
good, healthy hair and skin?

**ANSWER:** Health food. Preferably the kind that
never touches machinery. Natural food
—if possible, food that has been organically grown.

**27. QUESTION:** When hair has fallen out for several
years, due to ill health and hair dyes,
can it and will it grow in abundantly
again?

**ANSWER:** Yes, I certainly believe it can. But it is
not done simply by wishful thinking
on your part. You must help. Go to
your refrigerator and throw out all the
junk foods. Go to your cupboard and
clean out the senseless foods. Go to
your bathroom and remove the hair
dyes from the medicine chest or wherever you are hiding them. Cancel the
next appointment at the beauty salon
if that is where they try to make you
look younger every Friday. Go to a
health food store or worthwhile market
and actually buy some strange, myste-

rious health foods. Your family's hair is at stake as well as your own. Make the job of keeping your hair healthy a family affair. Women, more than men, control the health within a family by the way they shop—and the manner in which they cook. Most women, 99 percent of them, do not know how to boil an egg, how to protect the egg's fertility, hormones, and vital nutrients.

**28. QUESTION:** What do you think of massaging the whole body with oil?

**ANSWER:** I approve of the massage part, but what are you trying to accomplish with the oil? The skin should be oiled inside-out. The only real reason anyone should oil his skin outside-in is perhaps for suntanning purposes. I find that a good grade of baby oil applied liberally to the entire body, incidentally, will help you get a beautiful suntan. Some sun worshipers have told me that by adding a few drops of medicinal iodine, the combination can be even more effective for suntanning. But start at five minutes per day under a sun lamp and increase very gradually. Keep goggles or wet absorbent cotton over your closed eyes.

**29.** QUESTION: Should soap be used on the face?

ANSWER: There are other ways, but I believe soap will clean the face best. I use a soap that is enriched with lanolin.

**30.** QUESTION: Is very hot and very cold water good for the face?

ANSWER: I don't know. I use lukewarm water only.

**31.** QUESTION: What is the best shampoo and rinse for the hair?

ANSWER: A soapless shampoo and a high-quality organic rinse. These can be found in most health food stores.

**32.** QUESTION: Do you recommend the use of vinegar?

ANSWER: On a salad, yes, along with oil. In a drink, *no!*

**33.** QUESTION: What to do for gray hair?

ANSWER: I would leave it alone. I wish I had a head full of gray hair! I think anyone with 500 blond or black hairs, for example, would exchange them for 100,000 gray hairs. What you should do is to learn how to make your gray hair lustrous by adopting proper eating habits. Clean, dandruff-free gray hair is attractive whether in a man or a woman.

**34.** QUESTION: Is there anything that can make hair grow thicker or heavier?

ANSWER: I improved my hair with raw wheat

germ oil, raw wheat germ, and raw, organic onion. Other germinating foods and other measures also helped me, but I concentrated on these three food supplements.

35. QUESTION: Is honey the same as white sugar?

ANSWER: No. You may use honey, but in moderation.

36. QUESTION: What makes gray hair take on a yellowish color?

ANSWER: Probably a combination of circumstances. The lack of pigment-producing factors in the bloodstream, some quirk in the diet, and probably too much sun.

37. QUESTION: Some people recommend a little lemon juice in a glass of water. Is this bad?

ANSWER: Neither good nor bad. If you like, drink it.

38. QUESTION: Are hair and nails dead or alive?

ANSWER: They are very much alive—at the base. Dead at the ends.

39. QUESTION: Can you explain why the type of eggs you recommend helped you grow hair?

ANSWER: They're fertile. But growing hair is an art; it is not easy. The eggs merely assist the diet program.

40. QUESTION: How can thinning hair be restored when no excessive amount of dandruff is present?

ANSWER: All it takes to start hair falling is a little, teeny bit of dandruff. Dandruff is a red flag warning that the diet is faulty.

**41.** QUESTION: Is wheat germ oil the only dietary oil that can be helpful in a hair rehabilitation program?

ANSWER: Although wheat germ oil is the best oil you can take during your hair recovery program, it's quite all right to use other dietary oils. For instance, you may eat salads to which an oil and a little vinegar, preferably apple cider vinegar, has been added.

# 16

# LET'S GET STARTED ON YOUR HAIR—SAVING PROGRAM NOW

Don't be one of those well-intentioned but lazy people who put off getting started on anything until they forget it.

You now have all the basic information I ever had when I set out to avoid hair loss. The rest is up to you. If you begin taking the first steps toward a hair-nourishing program as soon as you finish this book, you may still save the hair you have left. You will also contribute to your general health. But you have to act soon.

Remember what I have stressed several times in this book. My program is designed to help grow back hair lost *within the last five years*. This means that the longer you wait, the less chance you have of reaching your goal. It finally dawned on me that if I wanted to have a healthy, lustrous, handsome head of hair, I had

199

to let the germinating foods begin their work before more damage was done to the precious hair seeds. Every day that you eat the wrong foods, especially hair-destroying foods like white sugar and other sweets, you are killing hair that might be saved by a change in your dietary habits.

It's not going to be easy at first. I'm quite aware of that. Our bad eating habits cling to us like leeches. It takes a great deal of willpower to change them, and the temptation to fall back on the wrong foods is always there. The tasty sweets, the fried foods, the heavily salted snacks sing their siren song wherever you go. If you watch television, the siren songs almost convince you that nothing else edible exists.

If you're a typical American, you eat copious quantities of potato chips, fried hamburgers, soft drinks, ice cream, cakes, and pies. Your medicine cabinet is probably well supplied with the more popular hair groomers and conditioners and soapy shampoos. And if you're a typical American, your hair continues to fall out.

You may be worried about your receding hairline or the increasingly large bald patches on your scalp. So what are you doing about it? You're probably trying one of the many greasy and alcoholic panaceas on drugstore shelves. And I'm sure your hair is still falling out. The greasy kid stuff from the druggist is doing nothing but lubricating your outer hair. Scalp clinics are another matter. They can and do contribute something positive in the way of massaging, stimulating, and cleaning your scalp. But they are only treating your problem *externally,* and it is my experience that hair problems must be treated *internally* as well. The condition of your hair is basically an *internal problem.* Never forget that!

You must think of your scalp, as you should indeed of your whole body, as a house that has a good foundation but is lined with lead pipes instead of copper plumbing. Within a reasonable span of time, ordinary water will corrode these pipes. In a similar fashion, sugars, fried foods, salts, and the like will corrode your hair follicles. To keep a house in good condition requires constant attention. Sun, wind, rain, and snow chip away at the house day after day. In a similar fashion, bad foods take their inevitable toll of your hair and scalp.

You do no tangible damage with one bag of salty, roasted peanuts or one bag of greasy potato chips. You don't kill your hair with one dish of ice cream or one soft drink. But if you persist in consuming foods that have been doctored to taste sweet or tangy or piquant, then these foods in time will have their inevitable effect on your health—and not just on your hair alone.

If you want to arrest your baldness and your dandruff, then you must tell yourself every time you eat:

"I am putting food into the bloodstream that will affect my health in general and my hair in particular for better or for worse. Do I want to injure my health and my hair or do I want to enhance them?"

You must determine now to add properly selected

foods to the bloodstream. You must stick to such foods. An occasional lapse will not matter. You can still have a soft drink or a hamburger or a few potato chips upon occasion if you must. But no more than occasionally. The emphasis must be on the right foods that will benefit not only your hair but your entire body.

It will help if you keep the image of the healthy Hunzukuts before you. Remember that tribe in Asia where men live to be 120 years old and are sexually potent at ninety? Keep in mind that these men who have heads of healthy, lustrous hair when they are over 100 eat only natural, unadulterated foods. Remember the Hunza diet: millet, barley, wheat, buckwheat, fresh organically grown vegetables, mutton, cheese, butter, and milk. And remember that there are only two bald men among the Hunzukuts—the two who acquired bad eating habits in England.

### Lazy Men Won't Try the Diet

I have learned from sad experience that the lazy man will not attempt the diet. Perhaps it was his laziness and negligence that caused his hair problem in the first place. Unless such individuals overcome their sloth, there is little help I can offer them. This diet takes exceptional discipline and willpower.

Many other balding men have to overcome a cynicism that has been caused by too many failures. This is something I can well understand. They have ransacked the shelves of pharmacies for a wonder drug or pill to bring their hair back. Everything they've tried has failed. It is understandable that these men should be skeptical, and even cynical. To these men I say, You may well have failed because you were treating your baldness from the outside in instead of inside out. My diet may be the answer you have been looking for. Give it an honest try.

Finally, there are the balding men who claim to be well-adjusted to their baldness and who say they do not want to do anything about it. But I have found that when you talk to them at any length, they usually confess their unhappiness. They are not really very secure with their hairpieces, and even less so without them. I am convinced, after many interviews, that no bald or balding man exists who does not want to re-grow his lost hair. Anyone who denies that is fooling only himself.

One more point: while I keep referring to "balding men," let's remember that even teen-agers sometimes suffer from early loss of hair.

## Don't Procrastinate

Once you have decided to do something about your loss of hair, you should act at once. Stop eating the wrong foods and get on to the right ones—today.

You have no time to lose. Remember that the rate of hairfall is always highest at the beginning.

Stray from the diet as little as possible. Remember, too, that the longer you stay on it past the 150 days the hair cycle takes, the more likely it is that you will grow back hair lost within the last five years.

Keep in mind the other things you must do, along with eating the right foods. Keep your scalp clean with a soapless shampoo, brush your hair regularly, and massage your scalp as directed.

Stay away from drugs and pills as much as possible. Take proper exercise so that your circulation is good and your body can do a good job of eliminating its poisons. In the language of the astronauts, all systems should be *Go*.

Start by opening your refrigerator and tossing out all the junk foods that are identified in this book. Then clear out the culprits in your pantry. When that's done, throw the descendants of the hippo fat remedy out of your medicine cabinet. And *now*—start on the hair-nourishing program outlined in this book.

I've now done all I can for you. The rest is up to you!

# INDEX

## ABOUT THE AUTHOR

DALE ALEXANDER is the author of the bestselling *Arthritis and Common Sense,* which sold more than 800,000 copies in its hardcover edition. It was while lecturing on his book on arthritis, and while discussing the diet he perfected to help arthritics, that the idea came to him to tackle his own problem — and that of millions of others — of approaching baldness. This book is the result of many years of intensive personal research and medical investigation.

### "Send a copy of this book to a friend"

All of us know many people who are losing their hair. Perhaps you have a friend or relative who has this unsettling condition. Someone who would really appreciate receiving a copy of this book. Why not send a copy of HEALTHY HAIR AND COMMON SENSE as a gift? It's a sensible gesture—and you may be giving a new approach to a person who suffers from this situation. They will be grateful to you for years to come.

This page is to tell you that often Bookstores do not have this book in stock due to distributional problems. If after trying your local bookstore you are unsuccessful in locating it, then write directly to the publisher and they will mail you a copy immediately. The price is $7.95 plus 50¢ postage and handling. Just send your letters to

THE WITKOWER PRESS, INC.
Box 2296, Bishops Corner
West Hartford, Conn. 06117